Enhancement of learning: Does sleep benefit motor skill memory consolidation?

A DISSERTATION
SUBMITTED TO THE FACULTY OF THE GRADUATE SCHOOL
OF THE UNIVERSITY OF MINNESOTA
BY

Michael Robert Borich

IN PARTIAL FULFILLMENT OF THE REQUIREMENTS
FOR THE DEGREE OF
DOCTOR OF PHILOSOPHY

Dr Teresa Jacobson Kimberley, PT PhD

December 2010

UMI Number: 3434304

All rights reserved

INFORMATION TO ALL USERS
The quality of this reproduction is dependent upon the quality of the copy submitted.

In the unlikely event that the author did not send a complete manuscript
and there are missing pages, these will be noted. Also, if material had to be removed,
a note will indicate the deletion.

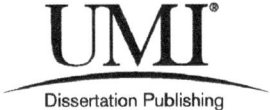
Dissertation Publishing

UMI 3434304
Copyright 2011 by ProQuest LLC.
All rights reserved. This edition of the work is protected against
unauthorized copying under Title 17, United States Code.

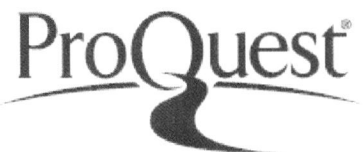

ProQuest LLC
789 East Eisenhower Parkway
P.O. Box 1346
Ann Arbor, MI 48106-1346

© Michael Borich 2010

Acknowledgements

I would like to thank the following individuals for their support, expertise and friendship: Tiffany Moore, My advisor: Dr. Teresa J. Kimberley, Dr. Kristen Pickett. Dr. Benjamin Clark, Faculty and Staff of the Rehabilitation Science and Physical Therapy programs, Dr. Michael Howell, Dr. Hartwig Siebner, Staff at the Masonic Clinical Research Center, fellow Rehabilitation Science doctoral students, Members of the BPL and my Committee Members: Drs. James R Carey, Paula M Ludewig, Juergen Konczak and Apostolos P Georgopoulos.

Dedication

This work is dedicated to my parents who have always supported me through everything. Without their love and support, I would never have made it this far.

Abstract

Purpose: It remains unclear how the brain best recovers from neurologic injury and how to optimally focus rehabilitation approaches to maximize this recovery. Recent research has indicated that sleep may augment this recovery. Sleep has been shown to benefit memory consolidation for certain motor skills, but it remains unclear if this relationship exists for explicit, continuous, goal-directed motor skills with rehabilitation applications. We aimed to determine the neurobehavioral relationship between finger-tracking skill development and sleep following skill training in young, healthy subjects. **Methods:** Forty subjects were recruited to receive motor skill training in the morning (n=20) or the evening (n=20). Measures of skill and cortical excitability were collected before and after training. Following training, each group had a post-training interval consisting of waking activity or an interval containing sleep. After this twelve-hour interval, skill performance and cortical excitability were reassessed. Subjects underwent another twelve-hour interval containing either waking activity or a sleep episode and came back for a second assessment, twenty-four hours after training. A subset of subjects (n=10) underwent the same procedures except the training period involved simple, repeated movement of the finger. **Results:** Skill performance improved after training and then continued to improve offline during the first post-training interval. Improvement was not enhanced by sleep during this interval. Cortical excitability was not substantially altered by training but was related to level of skill performance at follow-up assessment. Sleep quality was also found to be related to level of skill at follow-up assessments. The skilled training period did not lead to significantly improved performance compared to simple movement activity. **Discussion:** These data suggest that sleep is not required for offline memory enhancement for a continuous, visuospatial finger-tracking skill. These findings are in agreement with recent literature indicating the type of motor skill trained may determine the beneficial effect of sleep on post-training information processing. These results, combined with related studies in patient populations, provide a foundation to evaluate the relationship between sleep, changes in neural activity, and the time course of continuous visuospatial motor skill learning in individuals following neurologic insult.

Table of Contents

List of Tables	vii
List of Figures	viii
List of Appendices	x
Chapter I. Introduction	1
A. Defining motor learning and important factors in training paradigm design	1
1. Type and level of practice impacts learning	1
2. Feedback and learning	3
3. Task characteristics and motor learning	5
B. Memory categories and stages underlying learning	7
C. Neural basis of memory formation	8
D. Sleep and implicit memory consolidation	8
E. Sleep architecture: sleep states and memory consolidation	10
F. Qualitative and quantitative methods to evaluate sleep and sleepiness	13
G. Assessment of cortical excitability using transcranial magnetic stimulation	15
H. Preliminary work	18
I. Summary	19
Chapter II. Purpose	21
A. Hypotheses	22

	B. Research significance	24
Chapter III.	Methods	26
	A. Experimental design	26
	B. Subjects	27
	C. Instrumentation	27
	1. TMS targeting of M1 and cortical excitability assessment	27
	2. Visuospatial motor skill assessment	30
	3. Visuospatial motor skill training	32
	4. Movement activity	33
	D. Tests and measures	33
	1. Motor skill performance	33
	2. Cortical excitability	34
	3. Actigraphic sleep assessment	36
	4. Sleepiness and level of arousal	37
	E. Statistical design	38
	1. Power	38
	2. Statistical analyses	39
Chapter IV.	Results	42
	A. Finger-tracking performance in Day and Night skill training groups	42

B.	Measures of contralateral M1 cortical excitability	49
C.	Actigraphic assessment of sleep	54
D.	Relationship between tracking performance and subject characteristics	54
E.	Relationship between tracking performance and cortical excitability	55
F.	Relationship between tracking performance and sleep characteristics	56
G.	Effect of skilled tracking training versus repeated, simple movement	58
H.	Null hypotheses decisions	60
I.	Retrospective power analyses of results for primary H_os	61

Chapter V.	Discussion	62
A.	Summary of primary findings	62
	1. Sleep does not confer additional benefits to offline skill development	62
	2. Training did not increase measures of cortical excitability	68
	3. Sleep quality and skill development are related	72
	4. Tracking training did not increase tracking performance	75

Chapter VI.	Conclusions	78
Chapter VII.	References	79
Chapter VIII.	Appendices	89

List of Tables

1. **Measures of cortical excitability and proposed neural activity probed** — **16**
2. **Categorical list of dependent measurements** — **39**
3. **Demographic data: skill training groups** — **42**
4. **Demographic data: skill training and movement groups** — **58**

List of Figures

1. Tracking performance across assessments — 18
2. Relationship between change in tracking performance and SICI from pre-training to 24hr follow-up — 19
3. Schematic of primary research hypotheses organized by assessments for the skill training groups — 22
4. Schematic of hypotheses organized by assessments for skill training versus movement groups — 24
5. Research design — 27
6. Subject position for rMT and 1mVT determination — 28
7. Subject position for aMT determination and CSP measurement — 29
8. Subject position for finger-tracking assessment — 30
9. Target waveform used for finger-tracking assessment — 32
10. Examples of EMG traces during SP and PP data collection — 35
11. Example of EMG trace during CSP data collection — 36
12. Tracking accuracy for each S-R compatibility condition — 43
13. Tracking accuracy across trials — 43
14. Trial by assessment interaction for AI scores — 44
15. Accuracy index results between groups, across sessions, separated by S-R compatibility and trial — 46
16. Tracking lag across sessions between groups — 48
17. Accuracy and lag values between groups and training blocks — 49

18. SP MEP data across assessments, between groups	50
19. PP ratios across assessments, between groups	51
20. Resting motor threshold (rMT) across sessions	52
21. Active motor threshold (aMT) values between groups	53
22. One millivolt threshold (1mVT) values across assessments	54
23. Partial regression plots: tracking performance and paired-pulse MEP ratios at 12hr follow-up in both groups	56
24. Partial regression plots: tracking performance and sleep quality at 12hr follow-up in the Day group	57
25. Partial regression plots: tracking performance and sleep quality at 12hr follow-up in the Night group	57
26. Partial regression plots: change in tracking performance and sleep quality at 24hr follow-up in the Day group	58
27. Tracking performance across assessments between skill training and movement activity	59

List of Appendices

A.	Study consent form	89
B.	HIPAA medical information disclosure form	92
C.	Edinburgh Handedness Inventory (EHI)	94
D.	Sleep diary	95
E.	Actigraphic sleep scoring output example	96
F.	Stanford Sleepiness Scale (SSS)	97
G.	Pittsburgh Sleep Quality Index (PSQI)	98
H.	Epworth Sleepiness Scale (ESS)	100
I.	Example of normality and variance statistical outputs	101
J.	Example of univariate ANOVA statistical output	114
K.	Example of repeated-measures ANOVA statistical output	128
L.	Example of correlation and multiple regression statistical output	142
M.	Independent-samples t-test statistical output for demographic data	160
N.	Repeated-measures statistical output (trials 2-5) S-R compatible AI data	161
O.	Repeated-measures statistical output (trials 2-5) S-R incompatible AI data	165
P.	Repeated-measures statistical output for trial 1 S-R compatible AI data	170
Q.	Repeated-measures statistical output for trial 1 S-R incompatible	176

AI data

R. Change in AI from post-training to 12hr follow-up between training groups and tracking conditions — 181

S. Repeated-measures statistical output for trial 1 S-R incompatible tracking lag data — 182

T. Repeated-measures statistical output for mean (trials 2-5) S-R incompatible tracking lag data — 187

U. Repeated-measures statistical output for tracking performance during training — 191

V. Descriptive statistics for raw and log-transform single-pulse (SP) and paired-pulse (PP) MEP values — 197

W. Univariate ANOVA statistical output for SP MEP trial data — 198

X. Univariate ANOVA statistical output for PP MEP trial data — 208

Y. Repeated-measures ANOVA statistical output for mean PP MEP data — 212

Z. Repeated-measures statistical output for rMT data — 215

AA. Repeated-measures statistical output for aMT data — 218

BB. Repeated-measures statistical output for 1mVT data — 222

CC. Correlation statistical output for objective and subjective sleep quality and level of arousal data — 225

DD. Multiple regression statistical output: demographics/AI — 227

EE. Multiple regression statistical output: change in AI over — 230

	first 12hr interval/gender	
FF.	Multiple regression statistical output: PP ratios/AI at 12hr follow-up	232
GG.	Multiple regression statistical output: PP ratios/AI at 12hr follow-up, Night group	235
HH.	Multiple regression statistical output: TMS-evoked motor thresholds/AI at pre-training	238
II.	Multiple regression statistical output: Sleep quality/ S-R compatible AI at 12hr follow-up, Day group	246
JJ.	Multiple regression statistical output: Sleep quality/S-R incompatible AI at 12hr follow-up, Night group	249
KK.	Multiple regression statistical output: Sleep quality/ S-R incompatible accuracy at 24hr follow-up, Night group	253
LL.	Multiple regression statistical output: Sleep quality/change in S-R compatible accuracy across 24hr interval, Day group	256
MM.	Repeated-measures statistical output for AI: skill training versus movement	259

I. Introduction

Following neurologic insult, individuals often require extensive rehabilitation to regain their previous level of function. These individuals look to rehabilitation specialists to provide the expertise required to maximize their recovery. Unfortunately, full restoration of function is often not achieved. It is still unknown how the brain best recovers from injury and how to optimally focus rehabilitation approaches to maximize this recovery. Recent work has indicated that sleep may augment this recovery.

A number of theories have been put forth regarding the function of sleep ranging from energy conservation to synaptic plasticity enhancement (for review[1-4]). Sleep has been linked to memory formation for more than sixty years, but only recently have the neural mechanisms been investigated (for review[5, 6]). In particular, contemporary research has begun to illuminate the relationships between sleep and memory formation, including potential neural mechanisms[7-12]. If sleep is important for the memory formation underlying learning, then it is reasonable to assume that sleep could be important for rehabilitation following neurologic injury. Here, the salient aspects of learning and their influence on rehabilitation training paradigm design will be discussed. In addition, the underlying theoretical and neurobiological mechanisms involved in sleep and motor learning will be described leading to the primary unanswered research questions.

A. Defining motor learning and important factors in training paradigm design

Training paradigms consist of several important factors for rehabilitation and can significantly improve level and quality of recovery. In order to optimize learning rate and quality in both healthy and patient populations, these factors must be considered. These include: 1) type and level of practice, 2) performance feedback and 3) salient characteristics of a skill.

1. Type and level of practice impacts learning

Multiple studies have manipulated training paradigms to evaluate the effect of practice conditions on motor learning. In short, practice sessions that are variable and random tend to promote a greater extent of learning in comparison to constant practice of consistent variables[13]. Whether massed (within-trial time is greater than inter-trial interval) or distributed (within-trial time is less than inter-trial interval) practice is more beneficial remains unclear[14]. Also, the ability to generalize, or transfer, learning from one skill to another or between different environments is dependent on the similarity of the tasks and environments[14, 15]. Lastly, mental practice, either instructed by the trainer or independently generated, has been shown to improve performance on the rehearsed skill[16]. Each of these practice conditions must be considered in design of a motor learning paradigm either in a research or clinical setting to accurately evaluate outcomes and potential confounding factors to determine optimal training environments to maximize skill learning.

It has been argued that the most important factor in motor skill training is the amount of practice[13]. It has been shown that the rate of performance improvement is logarithmically related to the capacity for improvement[14]. In other words, the largest increases in skill are observed early during training and the rate of improvement diminishes over time although specific skill improvements can occur for years after initial exposure[14]. This relationship may explain the efficacy of short-term, intense rehabilitation paradigms including constraint-induced movement therapy and comprehensive acute rehabilitation programs.

Not only is the amount of practice important in motor learning, but also the delivery of practice. Based on the relationship between rate of skill improvement and time, it would appear that continuous, constant practice would be the preferred training method. Yet, other factors must be considered such as, fatigue, motivation and/or asymptotic performance with respect to time. It has been observed that over a training session, fatigue may occur either centrally or peripherally, which often leads to decrements in performance immediately after practice rather than expected improvements[17, 18]. In this case, performance improvements are often observed a short-time after practice has ended. This phenomenon has been termed, 'reminiscence', to differentiate from actual memory consolidation[17].

At a neuronal level, it appears that cortical plasticity is dependent on the activation history of a synapse. This has been shown in vitro[19] and in vivo[20, 21] where skill learning prior to cortical stimulation prevented long-term potentiation-induction while enhancing induction of long-term depression, the collection of synaptic processes underlying neuroplasticity and learning. This may be due to reduced neurotransmitter and receptor availability after learning. This may also provide a neural mechanism underlying asymptotic performance and fatigue associated with training. Therefore, it may be critical to provide intervals within and between training sessions to allow training-induced neurotransmitter and receptor changes on multiple levels to dissipate prior to further practice in order to maximize desired training effects.

At a neuronal systems level, it has been shown that cortical reorganization and skill learning are intimately related. This organization has been demonstrated by the expansion of the sensorimotor cortical representation of a limb after training[22, 23]. In contrast, when a limb is involved in repetitive, unskilled movement, reorganization does not occur[24]. Additionally, functional magnetic resonance imaging (fMRI) has demonstrated that skilled finger movement is associated with increased volume and intensity of cortical activation compared to an unskilled finger movement task[25]. Therefore, it can be hypothesized that changes in cortical organization and activity are dependent on the specificity and complexity of the task. Complex skill learning promotes lasting changes in cortical activity whereas simple, unskilled skill learning does not appear to significantly alter cortical behavior at a systems level. In order to maximize training-induced changes in behavior, choosing a task that is both relevant and complex is an important consideration in paradigm design.

2. *Feedback and learning*

During a training session, feedback is an essential component for modifying performance. It is apparent that the concept of feedback operates on multiple levels within the nervous system as well as across scientific disciplines from neuroscience to engineering[26]. In terms of motor control, feedforward and feedback mechanisms help shape motor outputs and can be influenced by the environment in which the system is behaving as well as the state of the system[26]. These mechanisms can be accessed during training by promoting intrinsic feedback and providing external feedback[27]. Intrinsic feedback is inherent to the behaving system and is usually thought of as the sensory information resulting from a movement. The information resulting from the combined feedback mechanisms provides a multimodal signal regarding the accuracy, or outcome, and quality of an action[28]. This signal can update an existing internal motor output model. Intrinsic feedback can also refer to the personal salience, or meaning of a given task, as well as the reward associated with successful production[13, 29]. In a neuroeconomical framework, it is argued that actions are selected based on the weighting of movement costs in comparison to expected reward[28, 29]. Costs and rewards can take many forms in this paradigm but put simply, a system will choose and refine actions that minimize costs and maximize rewards important to that system. In this framework, if a desired movement is inherently valued by an individual's reward system, this movement will be reinforced and is more likely to be produced when necessary. In the human nervous system, dopaminergic neurons are involved in mechanisms of motivation and reward within the ventral tegmental area as well as the network associated with movement production within the substantia nigra[30]. Relatedly, it has been shown that activity in the amygdala is associated with long-term memory formation further supporting the role of emotional context in memory formation[31]. This offers a physiologic link between reward and movement, supporting the role of intrinsic feedback in motor control and learning.

Feedback can also impact motor learning when offered externally either by the trainer or environmental response. Like intrinsic feedback, this information can also be multimodal and provided before, during and/or after skill production. Often, explicit extrinsic feedback is offered by the trainer regarding quality of movement, knowledge of performance (KP), or the outcome of a movement, termed knowledge of results (KR). Previous literature has focused on the optimal delivery of KR in terms of quantity and timing. It appears that this is also task-dependent with complex tasks benefiting from KR after five trials[32] while any KR minimally improves performance of tracking tasks[13]. However, it has been shown that constant, immediate feedback can actually have a detrimental effect on learning rate and/or capacity in healthy individuals[33]. It is hypothesized that excessive explicit information may overload the system taking up neural resources that could be used for other associated processes. In addition, it has been shown that explicit feedback actually can impair implicit motor performance in subjects with stroke[34-37]. Extrinsic feedback is a supplement to intrinsic feedback mechanisms and it appears that external conditions that promote motivation and reward provide the optimal means to enhance motor skill performance and learning.

3. Task characteristics and motor learning

Lastly, the components of a given motor task also influence the degree and mechanisms of motor skill learning. As mentioned above, conflicting results within the sleep and memory literature have not only been attributed to differences in research methodology but also to differences in task characteristics above and beyond the distinction of implicit/explicit information required and acquired[38]. Motor skills are often thought of as procedural skills that do not require substantial conscious cognitive involvement but it is clear that movement is a complex combination of implicit and explicit components[35, 39]. Research has attempted to control these interactions but even with carefully designed experiments, it still may be a limitation[40]. Explicit features of a task may include knowledge of: a goal to be attained in the paradigm, a desired movement and/or performance feedback. As discussed previously, explicit awareness impacts implicit memory consolidation[39]. Additionally, a motor task consists of implicit features that distinguish it from another skill. It can be continuous or discrete, complex or simple, single- or multi-joint or, closed or open.

The majority of skill learning literature has used an implicit version of the discrete serial reaction time task (SRTT)[41]. In this paradigm, subjects unknowingly acquire information regarding a repeated finger tapping sequence interspersed with random sequence trials[11, 42]. The difference in performance between these two conditions, after a task exposure period (training), is used to distinguish implicit learning from general improvements in movement efficiency[43]. Performance is usually measured by decreases in reaction time for the repeated sequence and, less consistently, number of sequences completed correctly[44]. Benefits of this research paradigm include: implicit components of motor skill learning are evaluated, outcome measures are simple and easy to interpret, and many functional skills consist of serial movements. Arguments against the SRTT include: lack of a continuous movement and outcome component, typically measure speed rather than accuracy and, extension of findings to most functional skills is limited due to lack of an explicit component.

Another common experimental paradigm focuses on dynamic adaptation learning. The experimental setup typically consists of subjects moving a manipulandum in a friction free environment to move a cursor on a computer screen from a start position to a target as fast and accurate as possible[45, 46]. Once learned, a force is applied perpendicular to the movement contingent on movement velocity. Path deviation and end-point accuracy are common measures of performance. This task differs from the SRTT in two important ways: 1) it requires explicit, online visual and sensory information and 2) outcome measures are continuous for the length of the trial, providing a measure of performance over time. These differences demonstrate functional relevance in terms of utilization of online internal and external feedback to modify movement to achieve an explicit goal. One disadvantage is that it only assays adaptation learning which has limited application to a vast repertoire of movements that may be (re)learned.

Lastly, skill learning has been probed using various tracking skills. Tracking skills can vary in many important ways but have two main components in common: 1) the task is continuous in nature and 2) performance is assessed over time using a continuous measure of error. Tracking skill can be implicitly-[47, 48] or explicitly-acquired[49, 50] depending on the type of sensory information provided. Visuospatial motor skill tracking training has been shown to improve functional outcomes and alter neural activity in stroke subjects when information is acquired explicitly and continuous visual feedback is provided[51, 52]. This specific task has also demonstrated off-line skill enhancement and is related to changes in cortical excitability in healthy individuals[53]. This task attempts to emulate components of a number of functional motor skills while maintaining sufficient experimental control to objectively investigate mechanisms involved in functional skill learning. Although this task has a number of advantages, it does not incorporate multi-joint movement and multimodal sensory processing is limited. Taken together, there are a number of components that can vary from one motor skill to another and interpretation of results should take these differences into account.

B. Memory categories and stages underlying learning

A primary challenge in sleep and learning research involves the application of various theoretical frameworks and computational models across multiple scientific disciplines to categorize and stage memory, the foundational principle of learning. A classical hierarchy for classifying memory types initially distinguishes between declarative and non-declarative information[54]. Declarative memories are consciously accessible and are divided into semantic and episodic sub-types[42]. Semantic memory refers to the knowledge of facts while episodic memory involves recollection of specific events[42]. Non-declarative memory is not consciously accessible and underlies the learning of actions, habits, and skills. Declarative memories are also commonly referred to as explicit memories while non-declarative memories are also known as implicit memories[38]. Classically, motor skill memories have been characterized by primarily implicit information and movement that does not require significant conscious awareness to complete successfully[55].

Stages of memory formation are usually expressed over a timescale beginning with initial information acquisition and memory encoding followed by memory consolidation that occurs over a time period following information exposure. Recently, consolidation has been reconceptualized into two subtypes: stabilization and enhancement[38]. During memory stabilization, an encoded memory becomes resistant to interference evidenced by a level of skill performance maintained over time that is not degraded with interference from information exposure[56]. Whereas, memory enhancement is indicated by not only maintenance of performance over time, but also by an improvement in performance without further task exposure[57, 58]. It has been argued that stabilization may be primarily time-sensitive while enhancement may be sleep-sensitive and task dependent[7, 12, 38, 59, 60]. These findings indicate that memory consolidation appears to be modulated by brain state of arousal and may offer unique opportunities to capitalize on the time- and task-dependent characteristics of skill learning.

C. Neural basis of memory formation

In order to examine the effect of various sleep stages on motor skill attainment, the underlying neural processes of normal motor learning and obligate memory formation must be understood. Synaptic plasticity is the neural basis of memory formation involving structural and functional changes in response to a given stimulus[5]. There are two predominate neural mechanisms involved in memory formation based on spatial and temporal parameters. Short-term motor memories are temporary, involve local synaptic modifications and need to be consolidated to persist over time[41, 61]. Long-term potentiation (LTP) and depression (LTD) of a given synapse results from altered pre-synaptic neuronal firing rates onto a post-synaptic cell[62]. When activity on both sides of a synapse is correlated, the synapse is strengthened, or potentiated[62]. When activity is uncorrelated or pre-synaptic firing rates are low, the synapse is weakened, or depressed[62].

Experimentally-induced potentation and/or depression have been shown to last for days to weeks from a given stimulus[63]. Synaptic strength can be altered by local changes such as pre-synaptic protein phosphorylation, retrograde communication as well as post-synaptic receptor density changes due to receptor and kinase phosphorylation[30]. If this activation is repeated and/or reinforced, short-term synaptic changes can lead to long-term synapse modification through altered gene expression and protein synthesis[30, 56, 64].

In motor learning there is a distribution of processing within the brain involving the frontal lobe motor regions, striatum and cerebellum which have been grossly linked by two distinct cortical-subcortical circuits: a cortico-striato-thalamo-cortical loop and a cortico-cerebello-thalamo-cortical loop[65]. These networks are reinforced and modified through plasticity of their synapses. Brain regions also demonstrate varied activation levels depending on stage of motor skill learning[66]. Local synaptic and cellular changes in each of these brain regions underlie motor skill attainment and are hypothesized to occur during periods of sleep[66-70].

D. Sleep and implicit memory consolidation

A considerable body of literature has supported a beneficial role of sleep in implicit sequence skill learning through enhanced memory consolidation[7, 9, 11]. Again, consolidation can result in stabilization of a newly acquired memory or even an enhancement of skill performance[39, 57, 60]. Explicit awareness of motor skill acquisition has demonstrated sleep-dependent performance gains that are not observed solely with the passage of time[39]. It also appears that sleep preferentially benefits goal-directed[57] and complex motor skill learning[11]. Most experiments to date have studied young, healthy, neurologically-intact individuals while only recently has motor skill learning and sleep been investigated in individuals post-stroke and age-matched controls [71].

Motor skills are comprised of multiple components dedicated to specific neural circuits[58, 72, 73]. Motor skills may develop after practice has ended, during a critical period of off-line memory consolidation, and sleep may benefit certain components of a recently acquired skill. Cohen and colleagues[57] have investigated this postulate using a variation of the SRTT where the movement (egocentric coordinates) component is disassociated from the goal (allocentric coordinates). This is accomplished by training one hand to perform a sequential tapping skill and then assessing performance on the contralateral hand where either the sequence remains the same, thereby requiring changes in finger movement, or the finger movements remain the same and the goal changes. This paradigm revealed that movement-based skill improvement occurs only during wake while goal-based enhancement requires sleep following training[57, 58]. These results further support a specific role for sleep in goal-directed motor skill development.

During motor sequence learning using the SRTT, it is difficult to control explicit information, or task awareness, thus limiting the ability to separate sequence learning from general skill learning[40]. Song and colleagues[40] addressed this issue by using a probabilistic SRTT paradigm in order to study the role of sleep on general motor skill and sequence-specific skill. The results demonstrated that sleep did not enhance general or sequence-specific skill learning, but skill improvement for general skill was found over an interval not involving sleep. Recently, these findings have been extended to a dynamic force field adaptation task[44]. This task requires the subject to move the cursor to a target using a manipulandum while a perturbation is applied during the movement. Performance on this task was compared to an explicit version of the four-element SRTT after an interval consisting of waking activity or one interval containing sleep. Results indicated that performance on the SRTT was enhanced following sleep while adaptation performance was improved with the simple passage of time[44]. These findings contrast previous sequencing and adaptation results by showing that not all motor tasks undergo sleep-dependent enhancement[74, 75]; however, these data may support a preferential role for sleep in enhancing explicit information associated with a given motor skill.

E. *Sleep architecture: sleep states and memory consolidation*

Sleep has been traditionally expressed as two distinct types: non-rapid eye movement (NREM) and rapid-eye movement sleep. NREM consists of four stages which vary in their electrical oscillatory properties observed by electroencephalography (EEG) and is thought to be a period of restoration and regeneration[38]. Recent studies have linked stage 2 NREM sleep to motor skill improvements in human subjects while others argue that stage 3-4 sleep consisting of primarily of slow-wave activity (SWA) is responsible for observed changes in neural activity and skill performance following sleep[7, 12, 76, 77]. Walker and colleagues[7] found that improvement of a sequential finger-tapping task was positively correlated with the subsequent amount of stage 2 sleep. Fischer and colleagues[12] conducted a similar study that differed on novelty of the sequential tapping task, and found performance gains were not related to NREM but, rather, to REM sleep. Stickgold and colleagues[77] reported early NREM sleep was associated with learning of a visual detection task, but Karni and colleagues[76] used the same task in previous work and found that NREM sleep deprivation did not impair memory. Currently, multiple studies have associated SWA observed in deeper sleep stages (0.5-4Hz) with memory consolidation[67, 70, 78-80]. These studies demonstrate the current state of literature regarding sleep stages and motor learning where conflicting results are common due to considerable methodological differences in study design and data interpretation.

Further support for a relationship between sleep and local cortical neuroplasticity has been provided by Huber and colleagues[67, 68, 70, 79]. Using transcranial paired associative stimulation (PAS), where medial nerve stimulation is paired with transcranial magnetic stimulation of the contralateral cortical representation of the hand, results have demonstrated LTP- and LTD-like changes in local cortical excitability depending on time between stimulations[70]. Subsequent sleep after PAS demonstrated local changes in sleep structure. Increased SWA, thought to be indicative of sleep need[81], was observed in regions of increased excitability and decreased SWA in depotentiated areas[68]. These findings were confirmed in a subsequent study[78].

The authors have also shown that arm immobilization, similar to constraint-induced movement therapy techniques, caused local decreased cortical excitability as well as decreased SWA in those specific regions[67]. Motor performance during a simple reaching task also deteriorated after immobilization[67]. Though specific levels of sleep will not be measured in this study, these findings demonstrate a relationship between motor skill performance, cortical plasticity, and sleep on a local level within the brain. Taken together, it appears that there is a significant link between induced changes in synaptic activity and observed changes in local cortical activity during sleep, evidenced by differences in oscillatory activity during certain sleep stages.

1. *Oscillatory properties of sleep may provide a mechanism for motor learning*

The rhythmic oscillations observed by EEG during NREM sleep demonstrate behavior that could promote synaptic modification. Thalamic oscillations result from concerted action potential generation due to coordinated Ca^{2+} and I_h channel activity which depolarizes the post-synaptic cell allows Ca^{2+} influx and causes prolonged after-hyperpolarization[82]. During stage 2 NREM sleep, these oscillations are referred to as spindles and occur at 7-14Hz. This activity initiates in the thalamus due to reticular system activity and projects to the cortex[83]. There is also significant cortical slow oscillation activity which has been found to be important in thalamic oscillation production and may provide a potential feedback loop[84]. As the thalamus is an integral portion of the primary motor loops as well as the cortex, there is potential for this rhythmic neural activity to influence motor skill consolidation through LTP and LTD as well as cellular modifications.

Slow oscillatory activity (0.5-4Hz) may also impact memory consolidation through synaptic depression or downscaling. LTD requires activation of a synapse without postsynaptic neuron action potential generation, which differs from LTP where both glutamate presence and post-synaptic depolarization are necessary. Low frequency stimulation (1-5Hz) of presynaptic inputs has been shown to induce LTD in animal models[19] and vary among brain regions[85]. Additionally, Marshall and colleagues[80] demonstrated transcranial application of low-frequency electrical oscillations during SWA sleep enhanced declarative memory consolidation but stimulation mimicking REM sleep was of no benefit. Tononi and Cirelli have found that molecules involved in depotentiation or depression are selectively up-regulated during NREM sleep demonstrating a cellular correlate supporting this hypothesis[3, 69, 86].

It has been argued that global downscaling of synaptic activity during sleep would improve performance by increasing synaptic signal-to-noise ratio[4]. This theory states that during motor learning, both efficacious and erroneous synapses are potentiated to different degrees. During sleep, global downscaling would reduce the strength of synapses by a proportional amount and weaker (erroneous) synapse strengths would become subthreshold and non-functional, while stronger (efficacious) synapses would be reduced but remain suprathreshold, thereby, allowing these synapse to remain viable[4, 87]. This may provide a mechanism to reduce unwanted noise and improve the signal of desired synaptic transmission[4, 87]. This hypothesis requires further investigation but does provide a testable framework on multiple levels of the nervous system to gain a comprehensive understanding of sleep-related synaptic plasticity following skill learning.

Although there is a strong theoretical framework and empirical data for the relationship of NREM sleep and motor learning, REM sleep has classically been linked with motor skill improvements[12, 76, 88]. Experimental data and theories have stated neural activity parallels waking and provides an environment to strengthen previously potentiated or further weaken depressed synapses[88]. This process could facilitate Ca^{2+} influx paired with post-synaptic depolarization thereby creating an environment for LTP to occur. It has been shown that visual-procedural memory consolidation is reduced when glutamate transmission is inhibited during sleep by administration of AMPA or NMDA receptor antagonists[89]. These results, paired with evidence supporting SWA and synaptic depotentiation, present a theoretical framework supporting complimentary roles for different sleep stages in the consolidation of recently acquired skills.

F. Qualitative and quantitative methods to evaluate sleep and sleepiness:

In humans, it is possible to evaluate sleep on multiple levels, from subjective report to sophisticated objective measurement. Subjective methods include self-report sleep logs or diaries and questionnaires regarding habitual sleep patterns, sleep quality and sleepiness, including: Pittsburgh Sleep Quality Index[90], Epworth Sleepiness Scale[91] and Stanford Sleepiness Scale[92]. These widely-administered measures have been shown to be valid and reliable in identifying cases of sleep disorders and responses to intervention[93]. These instruments are easy to apply and provide quantitative data regarding sleep-wake function. However, these data are not reliably related to objective measures of sleep[93]. Objectively, the gold standard for the measurement of sleep is polysomnography (PSG)[94]. This comprehensive approach measures the electrical activity associated with physiological changes occurring with different sleep/wake states in the brain (electroencephalography), heart (electrocardiography), eyes (electrooculography) and muscles (electromyography)[94]. It allows for quantification of sleep stages and is the primary tool for diagnosing sleep disorders. Although PSG provides excellent direct electrophysiological assessment of sleep, it is expensive, time-consuming, labor intensive and difficult to evaluate long-term sleep function in natural environments[95]. It also is often impractical to conduct PSG in research investigations or as a clinical screening tool[93].

A convenient, low-cost, easy to administer alternative to PSG for sleep measurement is actigraphy[96]. This methodology involves affixing an activity monitor, an actigraph, to the extremity or trunk of an individual[97]. The monitor uses an accelerometer to measure movement over time and is transduced into a digital representation[96]. This digital representation is known as an activity count and is subsequently subjected to a computer-based algorithm to determine sleep-wake activity[96]. This approach to assessing sleep-wake function is inherently limited by the indirect nature of the measurement but can provide useful data to allow for considered inferences of sleep quantity and quality[98].

Actigraphy has been shown to be strongly correlated with PSG in normal healthy adults[96, 99]. The sensitivity and specificity is lower in patients with sleep disorders [100] and does not correlate with PSG in critically ill patients, likely due to reduced movement during quiet waking that can be misinterpreted as sleep in this population[101]. The American Academy of Sleep Medicine practice parameters indicates actigraphy is a valid method to assist in determining sleep patterns in normal populations and certain sleep disorder populations, including insomnia and circadian rhythm sleep disorders[98]. Also, actigraphy has been included in the diagnostic criteria for, primarily, sleep pattern disorders in the second edition of the International Classification of Sleep Disorders[102].

Although actigraphy is simple to administer, there are several methodological challenges involved in data collection and analysis that may limit interpretation of results within and between similar studies. These include lack of uniformity in: data collection, analysis protocol, reporting of methodology, instrumentation, and selection of appropriate outcome measures[97]. Additionally, potentially significant sources of measurement artifact exist due to the uncontrolled environment in which actigraphy usually takes place[96]. Guidelines and recommendations have been put forth to improve the interpretability of the literature involving actigraphy in patient and healthy populations[96-98]. Advances in technology, increased research activity, and uniform study guidelines have made actigraphy a viable alternative to PSG to objectively quantify parameters of sleep patterns[98]. Yet, actigraphic assessment of sleep remains limited by an inability to directly measure electrophysiologic activity during sleep, instead, relying on inference of sleep-wake function from movement.

Actigraphy has been used in motor control and learning literature to a limited extent, usually serving as a control for movement when immobilization is desired[67]. It has been used to show that parameters of sleep are modified by physical activity interventions over long-term monitoring[103, 104]. Currently, there is a paucity of research evaluating the relationship between sleep patterns and motor skill learning. Based on the feasibility of actigraphy in research applications in comparison to PSG, it may provide a useful alternative approach to investigate the relationship between sleep and motor skill memory consolidation in larger sample sizes across an extended time course of measurement.

G. Assessment of cortical excitability using transcranial magnetic stimulation

Transcranial magnetic stimulation (TMS) is a non-invasive method to stimulate the brain[105]. This is achieved by discharging a high-voltage capacitor that is sent through a coil of conducting wire that induces a rapidly changing magnetic field[106]. When this field is applied over electrically-active tissue, it induces a transient change in current in adjacent tissue[107]. If this current is of sufficient intensity and applied over the scalp, it can cause an excitation, or depolarization, of cortical neurons[107]. This excitation is on a regional level, activating both cortico-cortical synapses as well as corticospinal efferent pathways directly[106]. If applied to the primary motor cortex, this excitation is quantified by measurement of the corresponding muscle response via electromyographic (EMG), recording termed a motor evoked potential (MEP).

A single-pulse (SP) MEP is a common measure of corticospinal excitability but is not specific to the cortex and requires parameter modification to identify the excitability of specific neuronal circuitry[108]. Single-pulse MEP amplitude often demonstrates a high degree of inter-trial and inter-individual variability that is reduced with increased stimulation intensity or muscle activation[106, 108]. This variability may also be due to coil position as small millimeter shifts and/or changes in coil orientation may change the induced electrical fields within the brain thereby altering the evoked response[109]. Thresholds for eliciting a motor response from a target muscle are identified by whether the muscle is at rest; resting motor threshold (rMT), 1mV threshold (1mVT), or active; active motor threshold (aMT) and, the level of EMG response indicative of a successful stimulation[110, 111]. These TMS-evoked stimulation thresholds are thought to represent cortical neuron membrane excitability[106].

A number of researchers advocate frameless stereotaxy using neuroimaging techniques to minimize the potential for this error[109, 112]. In many cases, logistical and financial constraints preclude the use of these multimodal imaging techniques and, therefore, coil localization remains predominately manual using the I0-20 International Electrode system to define cranial landmarks[106]. These landmarks have been found to be unreliable used in isolation but accurate stimulus localization is enhanced by systematically mapping the evoked response when stimulating areas within the primary motor cortex[106, 113]. Stimulation intensity/response curves are also used to address variability of MEP size[106, 108, 114]. This variability has been attributed to variable recruitment of motor neurons, variability in repetitive neuronal discharge and motor neuron de-synchronization[106]. Based on these limitations, single-pulse MEP is not an ideal single measurement of cortical excitability but may be used in conjunction with other excitability measurements to gain a comprehensive view of neural activity.

Additional techniques have been developed to measure excitability and changes in excitability in specific circuits, including cortical silent period (CSP) and paired-pulse short-interval intracortical inhibition/facilitation (SICI/ICF). The CSP refers to the cessation of voluntary activity of a target muscle in response to a suprathreshold TMS pulse. The latter duration of EMG quiescence during CSP measurement is reflective of the GABAergic activity within the stimulated cortical region[115]. In the paired-pulse technique, a sub-motor threshold conditioning pulse is paired with a supra-motor threshold test pulse at a fixed interval to measure intracortical synaptic activity[116]. When the interval is short (1-5ms), GABAergic function is targeted while longer intervals (10-15ms) target glutamatergic synapses[117].

Table 1: Measures of cortical excitability and proposed neurophysiologic locus

Excitability probe	Proposed neural activity probed
rMT	cortical neuron membrane, Na+-gated ion channels
aMT	cortical neuron membrane, Na+-gated ion channels
1mVT	cortical neuron membrane, Na+-gated ion channels
SP MEP	general cortiospinal activity
SICI	primarily intracortical GABAA-mediated synaptic activity
ICF	primarily intracortical glutamate-mediated synaptic activity
CSP	intracortical GABAB-mediated synaptic activity

These refinements in TMS instrumentation and application allow for decreased measurement variability as well as increased specificity of cortical excitability investigation. By combining measures of excitability, a multi-factorial assessment of neural activity can be conducted to further elucidate the neural mechanisms associated with behavior[106]. Although comprehensive measurement of cortical excitability can be made, conclusions regarding functional significance of these data can only be cautiously inferred due to the inability to directly assess cause-and-effect relationships between neural activity and observed behavior.

In addition to using TMS techniques to measure neural excitability, cortical excitability can also be modulated by TMS when applied repetitively (rTMS) in specific stimulus configurations. In particular, rTMS can be applied at varying discharge frequencies which have differential effects on cortical excitability[118]. When applied at a low-frequency ($\leq$ 1Hz), rTMS can inhibit cortical excitability while at frequencies greater than 1Hz, rTMS tends to facilitate cortical excitability[119, 120]. Low-frequency rTMS has been used to transiently inhibit neuronal activity, often described as a 'virtual lesion'[121], to assess contributions of a cortical region to a specific task[45, 122]. This approach affords the opportunity to non-invasively evaluate causal relationships between cortical activity and behavior[118].

Repetitive TMS has been used to investigate neural substrates of motor learning for a variety of tasks. Muellbacher and colleagues[123] investigated the effect of inhibitory (1Hz) rTMS after subjects were asked to perform repeated, externally-paced simple finger-thumb ballistic pinch movements. The acceleration used to produce the movement was assessed under multiple experimental conditions and demonstrated significant decreases in performance solely for those subjects receiving rTMS to M1[123]. These initial findings were replicated and also extended[45] to a motor adaptation task where subjects were asked to move their finger toward external targets in a null force field and then were exposed to a novel external force field. No decrement in performance was noted for the dynamic adaptation task when rTMS was applied to M1 after training in comparison to sham stimulation. This implies that motor memories for simple ballistic motor skills and dynamic skills may be distributed to different brain regions during immediate consolidation[45]. Other work has demonstrated implicit learning of a finger movement sequence was not affected by post-training rTMS application to M1 measured immediately after stimulation or after a 12hr interval containing sleep[60]. It did block off-line motor memory enhancement over an equivalent period of wakefulness[60]. Combined, these results demonstrate an integral role for M1 in initial motor memory consolidation of a ballistic skill, but it remains unclear if explicit learning of goal-directed tasks requires M1 for post-training memory consolidation.

H. Preliminary work

To investigate this question, we applied inhibitory rTMS to the contralateral M1 immediately following goal-directed, continuous visuospatial finger-tracking training and assessed changes in skill performance and cortical excitability[53]. We observed that tracking performance improved with training as expected but disruption to M1 did not significantly affect skill retention at 24hr follow-up assessment. In fact, all subjects demonstrated off-line memory enhancement indicated by improvements in skill performance post-rTMS compared to after training that were maintained at 24hr follow-up (Figure 1).

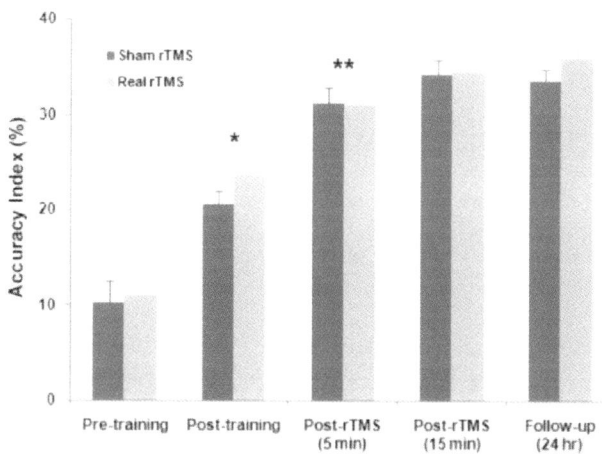

Figure 1: **Tracking performance across assessments (Mean ± SE)**. Tracking accuracy improved immediately after training (* $p<0.05$) and continued to improve up to 15 minutes post-

training (** p<0.05). These improvements were not attenuated by rTMS applied after training and were maintained up to one day following training.

Interestingly, we found a positive predictive relationship between the change in SICI and the change in tracking accuracy from pre-training to 24hr follow-up assessment. Before training, lower SICI values were associated with higher tracking accuracy whereas, at follow-up, this relationship was reversed. These findings suggest that cortical activity is modified over the time course of finger-tracking skill learning and may be due to off-line information processing occurring during the interval between training and follow-up. It remains unclear if waking activity and/or sleep contributed significantly to these observed changes in motor performance and cortical excitability.

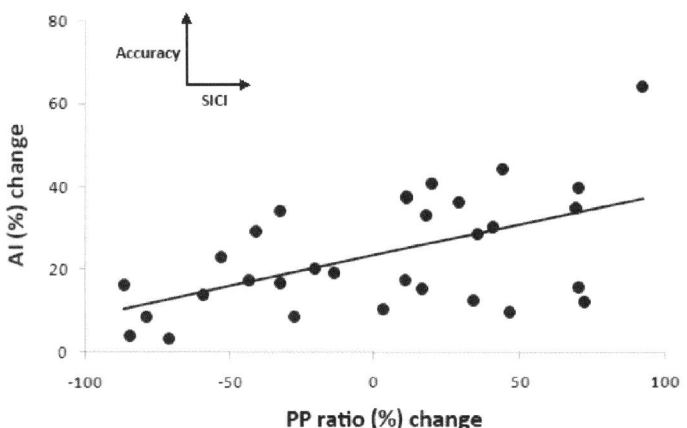

Figure 2: **Relationship between change in tracking performance and SICI from pre-training to 24hr follow-up**. Greater improvements in tracking accuracy were associated with increases in SICI, $R^2=0.27$, p=0.002.

I. Summary

The benefit of sleep in the learning of novel motor skills has been supported by a substantial body of research. It is believed that observed alterations in electrical activity, neurochemistry and functional anatomy during sleep compared to waking provide a unique environment for memory consolidation to occur. The causal contributions of specific sleep stages and characteristics are yet to be well-understood. Additionally, the benefits of sleep for motor learning have been predominately limited to motor adaptation and sequencing skill improvements in young, healthy individuals.

Non-invasive brain stimulation using TMS has become a popular method to investigate the neural substrates of human behavior. Using this technology, changes in cortical activity have been observed and induced under a vast number of experimental paradigms. Despite the intensity of inquiry, the relationship between sleep and motor learning with respect to cortical excitability has yet to be comprehensively understood.

In summary, there appears to be a relationship between sleep, motor learning, and neural activity but data are limited for functional skills that have 'real-life' functional significance to learning in healthy individuals and re-learning in people with neurologic injury.

II. Purpose

Previous work has demonstrated a beneficial role of sleep in the consolidation of memory for recently acquired motor skills, but it remains unclear if this relationship also exists for explicit, continuous, goal-directed motor skills that have direct applications to rehabilitation. Given the literature supporting a connection between sleep and motor skill performance, the purpose of this proposal was to investigate four principle aims:

1) Determine the role of sleep in the time course of memory consolidation of a novel visuospatial motor skill. Healthy subjects were trained on a novel, continuous finger-tracking skill during an initial session, either in the morning or evening. Tracking performance was assessed prior to, and immediately following training. After completing the initial session, both groups were assessed after twelve hours and again twenty-four hours after the initial session. One twelve-hour interval contained only waking activity and one twelve-hour interval contained an episode of sleep. The order of these two intervals was dependent on the time of day of the initial visit.

2) Determine the neural processes underlying motor skill learning as measured by cortical excitability in the contralateral primary motor cortex. For subjects in both training groups, cortical excitability was assessed before and after finger-tracking training during the initial session and after each post-training interval.

3) Examine the relationship between sleep quality and skill performance. Objective measures of sleep quality were collected for two nights: 1) before the initial visit and 2) either before 12hr or 24hr follow-up assessment depending on group assignment. Sleep quality during the night preceding skill assessment was used to evaluate the relationship between sleep and skill performance.

4) Determine the contributions of skill training to the time course of visuospatial motor skill learning. To address this aim, a subgroup of healthy subjects was asked to perform a simple, repeated finger movement during the initial session. The amount of exposure to this activity was equal to the skilled-learning training period. The research design for this group of subjects was identical to the skill training groups aside from the task.

The outcomes from this work aimed to make a significant contribution to the understanding of sleep and motor learning of a novel, continuous, goal-directed visuospatial motor skill. This improved understanding in healthy populations will facilitate future research investigations into the value of sleep for (re)learning motor skills following neurologic injury and the neurophysiologic mechanisms underlying restoration of function.

A. Hypotheses

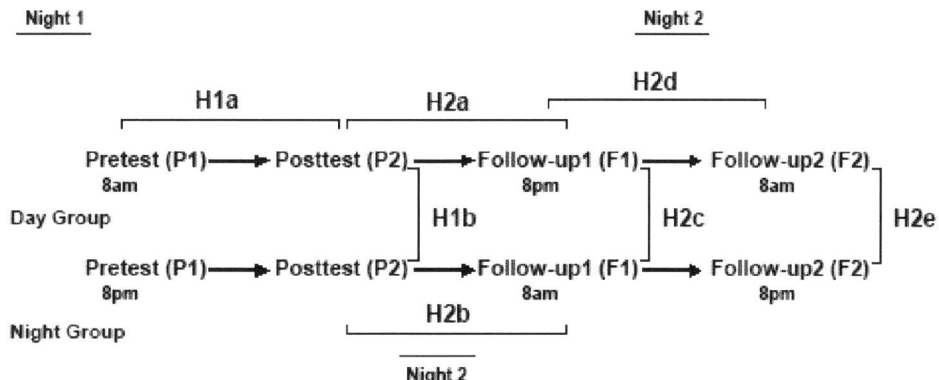

Figure 3. **Schematic of primary research hypotheses organized by assessments for the skill training groups.**

Based on previous literature, pilot data and research design, **it was hypothesized that:**

H1. Motor skill training **would** improve immediate skill performance.
 a. Following motor skill training, skill performance at P2 **would** be improved within groups compared to P1.
 b. Improvement **would not** be different between groups.

H2. Skill development **would** be dependent on first post-training interval.
 a. Following a waking interval, there **would** be significant skill improvement in the Day training group at F1.

b. Following an interval containing sleep, there **would** be significant motor learning improvement in the Night training group at F1.

c. These changes (H2a. and H2b.) **would** be affected by time of training evidenced by significantly greater performance improvement at F1 when the first post-training interval contains sleep compared to waking activity.

d. Within training groups, skill performance at F2 **would not** be different than at F1.

e. Skill performance at F2 **would** remain higher in the Night training group compared to performance in the Day group.

H3. Cortical excitability (CE) **would** be increased following skill training.
 a. Measures of CE (single-pulse MEP, paired pulse MEP, CSP duration and TMS-evoked thresholds) **would** demonstrate significantly increased primary motor cortex excitability within groups at P2, after finger-tracking training, compared to P1.

b. Measures of CE **would** be significantly reduced at both F1 and F2 compared to P2 within groups, but would not be significantly different from CE at P1.

c. Increases in CE following training **would not** be different between groups.

H4. Sleep quality and sleepiness **would not** be different between groups or testing sessions.
 a. There **would not** be a difference in sleep quality between groups for either night of sleep (N1 or N2).

b. Preceding night sleep quality **would** be positively associated with skill performance at P1 and F1 for Night group and F2 for Day group.

c. The relationship between sleep quality and tracking performance between training groups **would not** be different at any assessment.

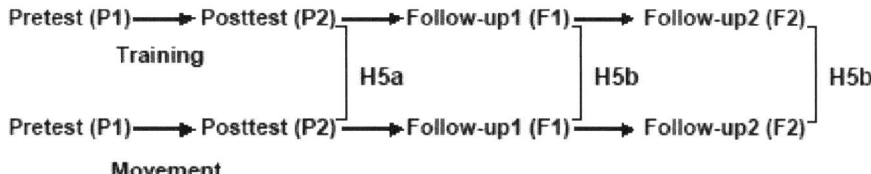

Figure 4. **Schematic of hypotheses organized by assessments for skill training versus movement groups.**

H5. Motor skill training **would** enhance skill performance in the training group but **not** the movement group.
  a. Motor skill training **would** significantly improve finger-tracking accuracy at P2 compared to unskilled, repeated finger movement.

  b. Finger-tracking accuracy **would** be significantly greater for the training group than observed for the movement group at both F1 and F2.

B. Research significance

This research provided a comprehensive evaluation of the role of sleep in the time course of motor skill learning and the neural mechanisms associated with this learning. This study aimed to build upon previous work demonstrating a beneficial effect of sleep for finger-sequence and adaptation learning by extending these investigations to an explicit, continuous, goal-directed, motor task. This work also attempted to evaluate the delayed effect of sleep on this task which had not been investigated previously. Additionally, this is the first study to examine the relationship between objective sleep assessment and motor performance over time. This study addresses important components of complex, functional motor learning that may have important future implications for multiple areas of rehabilitation.

The results of this work will provide a strong foundation for future studies investigating the therapeutic potential of sleep and sleep promotion on motor skill learning and neurologic rehabilitation programs.

III. Methods

A. Experimental design

A single-blind, pseudo-randomized design was employed whereby subjects were assigned to one of two age and gender matched groups (day skill training vs. night skill training). All subjects participated in three visits, each separated by twelve hours. During the first visit, subjects completed finger-tracking (FT) and cortical excitability (CE) assessments prior to, and following, one twenty-minute skilled finger-tracking training session.

The initial visit occurred either in the morning (n=20) or evening (n=20) based on group assignment. After a twelve-hour interval consisting of normal waking activity or an interval containing sleep, each subject returned for follow-up assessments of FT and CE without further training. After another twelve-hour interval containing sleep or waking activity, subjects returned for a second follow-up assessment of FT and CE, twenty-four hours after training (Figure 5). An additional group (n=10) was recruited to receive simple, repeated movement training that did not involve visuospatial tracking. In this group, all subjects began in the evening and the experimental design was identical to the primary design except for the training period. During the twenty-minute training, subjects performed repeated, unskilled finger movements rather than skilled finger tracking. During the 12-hour wake interval, subjects were instructed to refrain from napping. During the 12-hour interval containing sleep, subjects were instructed to refrain from alcohol intake or stimulant use to avoid changes in sleep quality and/or architecture associated with altered memory consolidation[124]. All subjects wore an activity monitor on their wrist during time in bed on the night preceding training and the night following training to objectively assess sleep quality[98].

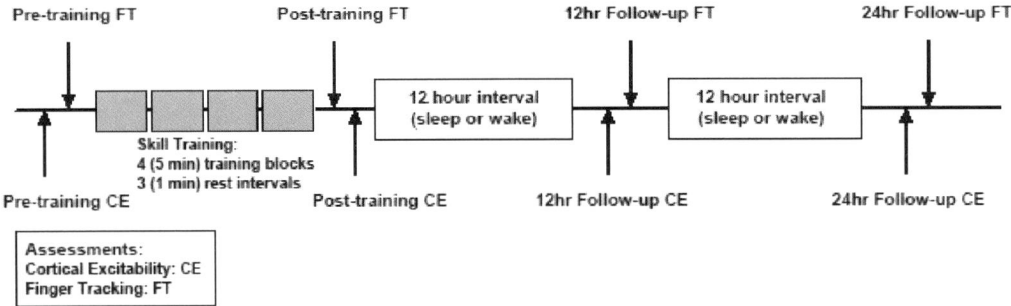

Figure 5. **Research design.**

B. Subjects

Fifty healthy subjects between the ages of 18-30 were recruited through the use of University and local community advertisement. Inclusion criteria: (1) 18-30 years of age, (2) right-handed, (3) no past history of neurologic disease, (4) no previous experience with finger-tracking activity, (5) no current orthopaedic impairment in right upper extremity and (6) normal joint ROM in right upper extremity. Exclusion criteria: (1) seizure history involving self or first-degree relative, (2) pregnancy, (3) metal in head (other than dental fillings), (4) implanted medical devices (pacemakers, medication pump, intracardiac lines) or (5) central nervous system-active medications. At the initial visit, all subjects gave written and informed consent (Appendix A) according to the Declaration of Helsinki. Following consent, subjects completed HIPAA medical information disclosure (Appendix B), inclusion/exclusion criteria was reviewed and study-specific questionnaires were administered (see Methods, Section D.3). Handedness was determined by the Edinburgh Handedness Inventory (EHI) (Appendix C)[125]. A physician (Dr. Sanjeev Arora) was available to examine each subject and review past medical history to ensure all safety measures were met and subjects were appropriate for participation.

C. Instrumentation

1. TMS targeting of M1 and cortical excitability assessment

Cortical excitability thresholds for the target muscle were determined using single pulse TMS targeted to the primary motor cortex (M1) contralateral to the test muscle. The resting (rMT) and active (aMT) motor thresholds were determined prior to cortical silent period (CSP) assessment. The 1mV threshold (1mVT) was identified prior to single-pulse (SP) and paired-pulse (PP) assessment.

While seated, subjects wore a tight-fitting Lycra swimming cap to mark the optimal scalp position for stimulation. Earplugs were worn by the subjects to prevent auditory threshold shifts and minimize stimulation-associated noise. Silver/silver chloride disposable electrodes were affixed in a belly-tendon montage of the right first dorsal interosseous muscle (FDI). To determine rMT and 1mVT, the arm was placed in a relaxed, comfortable position to minimize muscle activation in the limb (Figure 6). Alligator clip lead wires were attached to each electrode and connected to a Cadwell Sierra amplifier (Cadwell Laboratory, Washington) (sensitivity: 100μv/div, filter: 20-2000Hz). Electromyographic (EMG) signals were acquired at a sampling rate of 2560 kHz for 100ms, with a 10ms pre-stimulus epoch to monitor pre-stimulation activation to ensure the muscle remained at rest. For aMT, subjects were asked to actively abduct the second digit (5-10% of maximum voluntary contraction of FDI[126]) against a strain gauge coupled to a load cell (Figure 7). Continuous visual feedback of contraction level was provided on a computer screen in front of the subject.

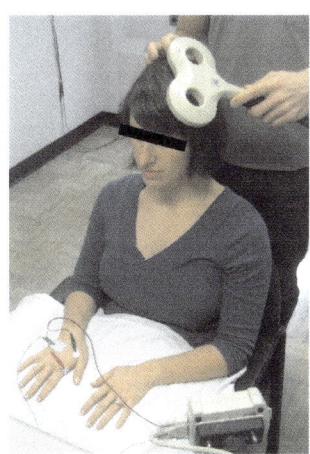

Figure 6. **Subject position for rMT and 1mVT determination.** Same position was used for single- and paired-pulse assessment.

To find the optimal position for activating the FDI, a 70-mm figure-eight TMS coil connected to a Magstim rapid magnetic stimulator (Magstim Co Ltd. Dyfed, UK) was used. This coil provides increased stimulus focality and has been widely utilized to stimulate cortical tissue with a maximal depth of penetration of ~25mm[107, 127]. The coil was held tangentially to the skull with the handle directed 45° posterolateral to the midsagittal line of the skull over the approximate area of M1 in the contralateral hemisphere and moved systematically to find the optimal position. This orientation has been shown to optimally target descending cortical axons in the stimulated region[106, 109].

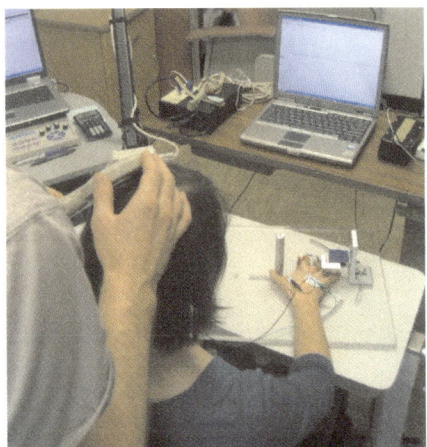

Figure 7. **Subject position for aMT determination and CSP measurement.**

Single-pulse magnetic stimuli were delivered manually to the scalp location overlying the presupposed M1 locus for optimal FDI activation at approximately 0.1 Hz starting at an intensity of 50% of the maximum stimulator output. For rMT determination, level of intensity was adjusted systematically until the rMT was found, defined as the minimum intensity required to elicit MEPs >50 µV peak-to-peak in at least 5 of 10 trials of FDI at rest[110]. Once intensity was identified, the location of coil was systematically moved 1cm anteriorly, posteriorly, medially and laterally to assess responsiveness of neighboring regions to stimulation. The final location was then used to determine intensity level of aMT and 1mVT. The same procedure was used for aMT determination except the MEP elicited had to exceed 200μV peak-to-peak in at least 5 of 10 trials[110]. For 1mVT, stimulus intensity was varied until MEPs of ~1mV were consistently evoked[111]. Using these identified intensities, cortical excitability was assessed utilizing the measures outlined below. These measures were collected before and after training, at 12-hr follow-up and, at 24-hr follow-up.

2. *Visuospatial motor skill assessment*

To investigate motor skill performance, subjects were tested on a novel finger-tracking task involving flexion and extension movements of the right index finger. A custom-made electrogoniometer, consisting of a potentiometer attached to a splint, was used. When donned, the potentiometer was centered at the index finger metacarpophalangeal (MP) joint to measure change in joint position during active movement[128]. The electrogoniometers have been found to be accurate to within 1 degree over a 120-degree range [50]. The forearm was placed in a pronated position for testing and supported while allowing full index finger ROM. In addition, the shoulder was allowed to rest comfortably at the side with the elbow at ~90° of flexion (Figure 8).

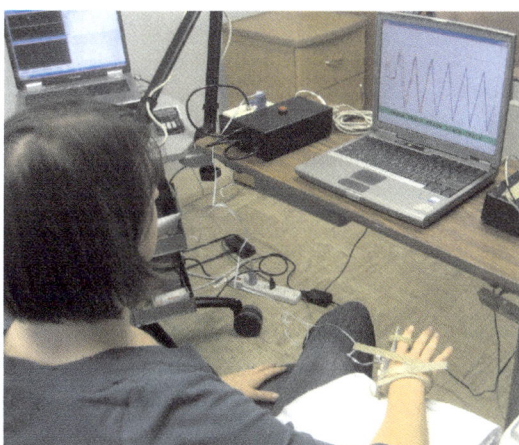

Figure 8. **Subject position for finger-tracking assessment**. The same position was used for the training protocol.

Active movements involved tracking of a computer-generated target waveform moving independently at a fixed frequency from left to right on a computer display in front of the subject. Modifying target parameters and tracking conditions creates varied contexts for goal-directed movement[128]. First, maximum flexion and extension excursion was assessed for each subject to account for individual range of motion (ROM) differences. After, subjects were verbally instructed on the goal of the tracking task as well as the dynamics of the task. Then, their finger was passively moved during one 5-second practice trial. During another 5-second trial, subjects actively tracked the target to ensure task familiarization while maintaining task novelty.

During each FT assessment, there were ten consecutive 10-second tracking trials presented. Half of the trials were stimulus-response (S-R) compatible and the other five were S-R incompatible. In the compatible condition, the cursor moved in the same direction as finger movement while in the incompatible condition, the cursor moved in the opposite direction of finger movement. These two conditions were randomly presented during each FT assessment. The test waveform was a triangle wave with a peak-to-peak amplitude of 15%-85% of each subject's full, comfortable ROM (Figure 6). The tracking cursor moved from left to right across the computer screen placed at eye-level, ~60cm from the subject, at a frequency of 0.6Hz. These parameters were chosen based on rapid skill acquisition for this waveform[129] and pilot data demonstrating substantial offline skill enhancement over 24hrs following training with reduced variance compared to other waveforms between subjects (n=4). The training protocol began immediately following completion of the first FT assessment and the post-training FT assessment was completed directly following the end of the training protocol. The FT assessment was then repeated 12 and 24 hours after training completion.

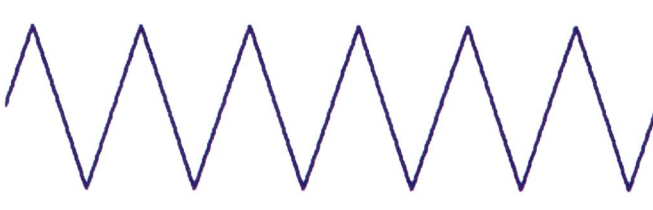

Figure 9: **Target waveform (blue) used for finger-tracking assessment.**

3. Visuospatial motor skill training

The same tracking apparatus and positioning used for FT assessment was utilized for the 20-minute motor skill training session. This training consisted of 105 trials separated into four 5-minute training blocks with 1-minute rest periods between each block to minimize fatigue and promote optimal effort and motivation. Knowledge of performance was provided by a cursor trace produced during each trial but no feedback was given by the examiner to control for potential differences in feedback quantity and/or quality. Knowledge of results (KR) was provided every fifth trial in the form of an accuracy score displayed after trial completion for one second during the first two training blocks. In the third and fourth blocks, KR was faded and provided every tenth trial. For each 5-minute training block, there were 27-30 trials with a one second rest in between each trial.

A host of training protocols, created by varying tracking conditions and target parameters, were used to introduce variability and promote greater depth of cognitive processing. These variations included: altering peak-to-peak amplitude of finger movement (0-100% of individual ROM), frequency (0.2-1.0Hz), adjusting trial length (5-20 seconds), changing the target waveform shape (sine, cosine, sawtooth, square, random), reversing potentiometer polarity to introduce stimulus-response incompatibility[130] and modifying forearm position (full pronation or neutral). The task employed during the skill assessments described above was not repeated in the training protocol to avoid practice-related improvements on the test waveform outside skill assessments. This training paradigm was identical for all subjects.

4. *Movement activity*

To determine performance changes associated with motor learning following finger-tracking training vs. movement alone, a repetitive movement exposure session was administered to a subgroup of subjects (n=10). Subject positioning and tracking apparatus were identical to the skill training group. The number of trials and trial blocks within the session were also identical. During each trial, a cursor swept across the screen but the target and response were not shown[52]. Subjects were instructed to perform repeated flexion/extension movements of the right index finger within 80% of their available ROM at an approximate frequency of 0.4Hz. Movement velocity was paced by a metronome timed at 44bpm and subjects were instructed to complete one flexion or one extension movement during each inter-beat interval. This frequency was determined by averaging the frequencies of all the trials in the skill training group in order to control for movement velocity and absolute number of movements of the index finger. Movement amplitude, frequency and velocity were monitored by study staff throughout the 20-minute movement session. These parameters were intended to minimize kinematic differences between the skill training and movement groups that can affect cortical activation[131].

D. *Tests and Measures*

1. *Motor skill performance*

Motor skill performance was measured by tracking accuracy and lag. Tracking accuracy was represented by an accuracy index (AI): AI= $100(P-E)/P$ where E is the root-mean square error between the target line and the performance line and P is the size of the target pattern defined as the root mean square difference between the wave and the midline separating the wave[128]. This measure has been previously validated in healthy and stroke populations[50, 132]. This accuracy value accounts for inter-subject differences in finger ROM to determine individual tracking performance and compare across subjects. Tracking lag assesses the degree in which the response trails the target in the time domain. It is computed by measuring the peak cross-correlation between target and response. Tracking lag primarily assesses the temporal aspects of skill performance while AI depends both on the spatial and temporal aspects of performance. It has been argued that different aspects of a skill may undergo different mechanisms of consolidation during post-training learning[133].

2. *Cortical excitability*

Cortical excitability was assessed through four measurements: 1) Single-pulse (SP) MEPs, 2) Paired-pulse (PP) MEP amplitude (3ms/10ms), 3) cortical silent period duration and 4) motor threshold stimulation intensity (rMT, aMT, 1mVT). Each measure collected is thought to probe a specific neural contribution to cortical excitability.

1) Single-pulse MEPs were collected at a stimulation intensity found to evoke a consistent ~1mVT response from FDI during threshold determination. Ten trials were collected prior to PP MEP collection and then ten trials were obtained after PP assessment (gain: 500μv/div, filter: 20-200Hz, sweep interval: 10ms/division). Peak-to-peak amplitude was identified for each MEP collected (Figure 10). By collecting SP MEPs before and after, potential priming effects of PP stimulation protocol were minimized.

2) Paired-pulse MEPs were collected to assess short-interval intracortical inhibition (SICI) and intracortical facilitation (ICF), where a subthreshold (90% aMT) conditioning pulse was delivered at a short (3ms) or long (10ms) interstimulus interval (ISI) prior to suprathreshold (1mVT) test pulse delivery (Figure 10)[116, 117]. Paired TMS stimuli were delivered with two Magstim 200 devices connected through a Magstim BiStim^2 Module (Magstim Co LTD, Whitland, UK) through a standard 70-mm coil over the previously identified location of FDI activation while the hand was at rest. The test pulse intensity was chosen to avoid ceiling or floor effects associated with the conditioning pulse[111]. Ten trials were collected for each ISI alternating between ISIs every two trials to minimize priming effects.

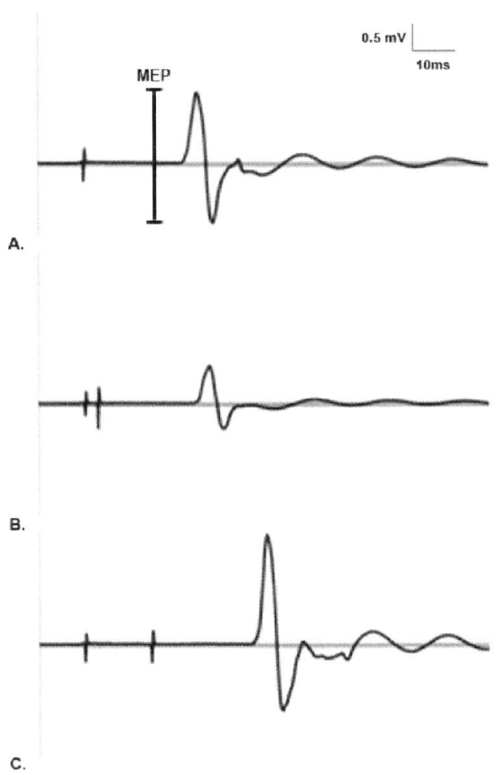

Figure 10. **Examples of EMG traces during SP and PP data collection**. A) SP MEP, B) PP MEP, ISI=3ms, C) PP MEP, ISI=10ms.

At each assessment, ten MEPs were obtained for each inter-stimulus interval (3ms or 10ms). Again, peak-to-peak amplitudes were measured for each MEP collected. These data were then indexed to the mean SP MEP amplitude (n=20 trials) for the same assessment session (PP MEP/SP MEP$_{\bar{x}}$)[134] in order to assess the conditioning pulse effects on the MEP amplitude evoked from the test pulse.

3) To determine cortical silent period (CSP) duration, subjects performed a sustained abduction force (20% maximum voluntary contraction) of the index finger against a strain gauge coupled to a load cell. Force output was transduced and displayed on a computer screen placed in front of the subject. Subjects were asked to maintain this contraction for 6 seconds while a single magnetic pulse (150% aMT) was administered. Trials were collected every 20 seconds to prevent fatigue

and summative effects of the stimulation. To determine CSP onset, the first superimposed TMS-induced EMG peak was identified. The CSP offset was defined as the resumption of sustained volitional EMG activity that surpassed 50% of the average prestimulus EMG activity (25ms). This scoring method has been shown to be reliable in healthy subjects and patients with focal hand dystonia[135] (Figure 11).

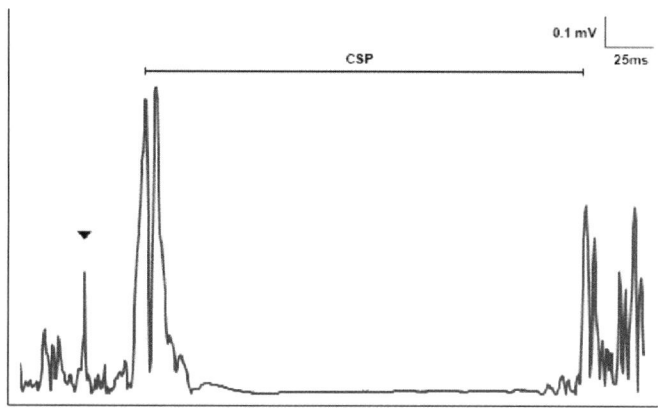

Figure 11. **Example of EMG trace during CSP data collection**. Triangle denotes stimulus artifact.

4) Determination of motor thresholds was described above and repeated at each assessment prior to data collection of the above measures of cortical excitability.

3. *Actigraphic sleep assessment*

Subjects wore an activity monitor (ActiSleep sleep monitor, ActiGraph™, Pensacola, FL) on their wrist during the night before beginning the experiment and during the night after training. Subjects were instructed to wear the monitor on either dominant or non-dominant extremity but to use the chosen extremity for both nights. Subjects also completed a sleep diary for each night (Appendix D). Movement data was collected, summated over 60-second epochs and converted to digital activity counts at 60Hz. Sleep scoring was conducted using the ActiLife software package (v. 4.4.1, ActiGraph™,

Pensacola, FL). An adapted scoring algorithm was used to determine the sleep state for each recorded epoch across a sliding 11-minute window. The algorithm has previously demonstrated >90% agreement with polysomnography for sleep-wake state determination[136]. The sleep diary was used to determine time into and out of bed. Measures of sleep were: (1) *sleep onset (min)*: Indicated by the first activity epoch determined to be "asleep"; (2) *time asleep (min)*: The time between sleep onset and final awake time; (3) *sleep latency (min)*: the time between time-into-bed and sleep onset; (4) *awakenings (#)*: the number of different times determined to be "awake"; (5) *time awake (min)*: the total time determined to be "awake" during the sleep interval; (6) *average time awake (min):* time awake/awakenings; (7) *sleep efficiency (%)*: time "asleep"/total time in bed (Appendix E).

4. *Level of arousal and sleep characteristics*

Sleepiness and sleep quality were evaluated using the Stanford Sleepiness Scale (SSS)[92] Pittsburgh Sleep Quality Index (PSQI)[60, 90] and Epworth Sleepiness Scale (ESS)[91]. The SSS is a self-report scale rating current state of sleepiness and was administered at the beginning and end of the first session and at each follow-up session. It is a seven point scale (1-7) ranging from: 1=Feeling active and vital; alert; wide-awake to 7=Sleep onset soon; lost struggle to remain awake. This scale has shown a strong correlation with sleep onset latency[137] and been shown to be a reliable indicator of level of arousal[92, 138] (Appendix F). The PSQI is a 24-item questionnaire regarding sleep quality, duration of sleep, typical bedtime and wake-up time, sleep latency and frequency of sleep disturbances for the preceding month (Appendix G). The questions are separated into 7 categories, scored 0 (no difficulty) to 3 (severe difficulty). It has been shown to be valid and reliable measure of sleep quality with total scores above 5 indicating significant sleep disturbance[90]. The ESS is a measurement of general daytime sleepiness and subjects are asked to rate their likelihood of falling asleep while involved in eight different activities on a scale from 0=would never doze or sleep to 3=high chance of dozing or sleeping (Appendix H). The ESS has demonstrated high test-rest reliability and good internal consistency and is correlated with the Multiple Sleep Latency Test, considered to be the gold standard for objective quantification of daytime sleepiness[91, 139]. Values above 10 are considered as sleepy and over 18 are very sleepy[91]. The PSQI and ESS were administered to subjects in each group at the beginning of the first visit.

Data processing and quantification of all dependent measures were done by an investigator blinded to group assignment.

E. Statistical design

1. Power

Pilot work (n=4) investigating finger-tracking performance on the proposed test waveform following a 20-minute training session demonstrated a 9% improvement in AI between baseline and 24-hour follow-up testing. Combined with the greatest observed variance, SD=5.70%, 7 subjects/group were found to be required to detect a significant difference. In previous work comparing training effects of skill training versus unskilled movement training in subjects with stroke, a 25% difference in AI was observed between training paradigms[52]. Combined with the observed variance (SD=16%), 7 subjects/group were shown to be necessary to detect a significant difference between training groups. A power analysis based on a related study was used to determine the *n* necessary to detect a meaningful significant difference in goal-directed skill performance based on post-training interval[57]. In the study, significant differences in implicit finger sequence performance in the goal-based paradigm were demonstrated between over-day and over-night post-training intervals[57]. Based on measurement variability of SD= 47ms, the sample size required to have sufficient power to detect a meaningful significant difference (45ms) was 18 subjects/group.

For measures of cortical excitability, pilot testing (single-pulse MEP amplitude) in healthy subjects demonstrated that 13 subjects/group would be required to detect a meaningful difference of 125μV with a SD of 110μV. These sample sizes were derived from related investigations to this proposal but due to differences in methodology and limited sample sizes, a conservative estimate of sample size was considered, *n=*20 for each training group and *n=*10 for the movement subgroup. The same motor skill paradigm was used in our preliminary investigation with variations in study design and test waveform. Results indicated an n=16/sample was sufficient to detect significant offline changes in skill performance over a 24hr interval[53].

2. *Statistical analyses*

Normality and heterogeneity of variance were assessed for each dependent measure (Table 2) (Appendix I). If violations were observed, data transformations were attempted. If data was resistant to transformation, non-transformed data was subjected to parametric analyses based on robustness of statistical procedures[140]. Baseline differences in dependent measures between groups at pre-training assessment were evaluated using independent samples t-tests with training group as the grouping variable. Baseline differences in skill performance and cortical excitability were also assessed to determine if initial level of performance or excitability should be added to subsequent analysis steps as a covariate.

Table 2: Categorical list of dependent measurements

Outcome categories	Dependent measures	Abbreviation
Subject characteristics	Age	
	Edinburgh Handedness Inventory	EHI
	Pittsburgh Sleep Quality Index	PSQI
	Epworth Sleepiness Scale	ESS
	Stanford Sleepiness Scale	SSS
Motor skill performance	Accuracy index	AI
	Lag	
Cortical excitability	Single-pulse motor evoked potential	SP MEP
	Short-interval intracortical inhibition	SICI
	Intracortical facilitation	ICF
	Cortical silent period	CSP
	Resting motor threshold	rMT
	Active motor threshold	aMT
	1 millivolt threshold	1mVT
Sleep actigraphy	Sleep efficiency	
	Time awake	
	Time asleep	
	Average time awake	
	Awakenings	
	Sleep latency	

First, univariate ANOVAs were conducted to assess potential trial effects for each dependent measure with multiple trials collected during an assessment (Appendix J). If a significant main effect of trial or an interaction effect with group or assessment was observed, two-tailed post-hoc pairwise comparisons with Bonferroni adjustment were conducted. An additional within-subjects factor of stimulus-response compatibility (S-R compatibility) was added to the analysis of motor skill performance (AI, lag) to assess for potential differences in tracking performance between S-R compatible and incompatible conditions. For SP MEP, a factor identifying whether a trial was collected before or after PP MEP testing was added to the model to examine potential priming effects of the PP protocol. For PP MEP ratio data, a factor of ISI was included to evaluate the difference between 3ms and 10ms intervals between conditioning and test pulses as each of these intervals is thought to probe a different cortical pathway (SICI, ICF). Data were subsequently grouped based on these results and trials were averaged across each assessment for the next stages of statistical analysis.

Repeated-measures two-way ANOVAs with a main effect of assessment (pre-training vs. post-training vs. 12hr follow-up vs. 24hr follow-up) as the within-subjects factor and a main effect of group (day training vs. night training) as the between-subjects factor were conducted for motor skill performance (AI, lag) and cortical excitability (SP MEP, PP MEP ratios, CSP duration, rMT, aMT, 1mVT) measures (Appendix K). Interaction effects between group and assessment were also assessed. Repeated-measures ANOVAs were also conducted for actigraphy data with main effects of night (night before initial visit and night following training) and group. Mauchly's test was used to determine if sphericity was violated and, if violated, Greenhouse-Geisser adjustments to degrees of freedom were applied. Partial η^2 was calculated to determine the effect size of significant results. Levene's Test of Equality of Error Variances was used to assess dependent measure error variance across groups.

Secondary analyses using two-tailed post-hoc pairwise comparisons with Bonferroni correction for multiple comparisons were conducted for significant results. The same analyses were then used to investigate the differences in training activity (skill tracking training vs. simple movement).

Regression and correlational analyses were conducted to evaluate associations between dependent measures (Appendix L). Separate hierarchical multiple regression analyses were used to evaluate the predictive capacity of: 1) subject demographics (age and gender) on tracking performance at pre-training assessment and change in performance from post-training to follow-up assessments, 2) cortical excitability on tracking performance at each assessment, 3) objective measures of sleep characteristics (sleep efficiency, average time awake and number of awakenings) on tracking performance and change in performance from post-training to each follow-up assessment. For this analysis, the preceding night of sleep was used in the model. For example, at 12hr follow-up in the day group, actigraphy data from night 1 was used while in the night group, data from night 2 was incorporated. For each regression analysis, correlations between predictors and dependent measures were conducted first. Using these results and theoretical rationale, order of entry in the model was determined. Zero-order, part and partial correlations were produced for each model. Colinearity between multiple predictors was evaluated using Variance Inflation Factor (VIF) and Tolerance levels. Values under 10 for VIF and above 0.1 for Tolerance were critical levels for acceptable colinearity[141]. Residual statistics and plots were produced to ensure normality and heteroscedasticity of the data[141, 142]. Durbin-Watson diagnostics were provided to ensure independence of the residuals from the regression analysis. Casewise diagnostics were used to determine extreme outliers in the model (>3SD)[141]. Identified cases were removed and the regression analysis was run again. The final model for each analysis was based on overall significance of each model (critical α-level: p=0.05) and the significance level of the R^2 change when adding a new predictor to the model.

IV. Results

A. Finger-tracking performance in Day and Night skill training groups

1. Subject characteristics

Data were normally distributed and homogeneity of variance was confirmed (Levene's Test) for subject characteristics (age, gender, EHI, PSQI, ESS, SSS). There were no statistically significant differences for age, handedness, subjective sleep quality or sleepiness between day and night skill training groups (Table 3) (Appendix M).

Table 3: Demographic data

Group	Age	Gender	EHI	PSQI	ESS	SSS (pre)	SSS (post)	SSS (12hr)	SSS (24hr)
Day Skill	23.2 ± 3.9	M:10, F:10	74.4 ± 21.5	4.6 ± 2.3	6.7 ± 3.2	2.3 ± 1.1	2.3 ± 1.1	2.2 ± 1.3	2.4 ± 0.9
Night Skill	21.9 ± 3.8	M:10, F:10	77.7 ± 20.9	4.0 ± 1.8	7.9 ± 4.0	2.6 ± 0.9	2.7 ± 1.3	2.4 ± 1.0	2.1 ± 0.8

EHI: Edinburgh Handedness Inventory, PSQI: Pittsburgh Sleep Quality Index, ESS: Epworth Sleepiness Scale, SSS: Stanford Sleepiness Scale

2. Measurements of finger-tracking performance

a. Accuracy index (AI)

Accuracy index data were not found to violate the assumptions of normality. First, to evaluate the main effects of stimulus-response (S-R) compatibility and trial on AI, a univariate four-way (group by assessment by S-R compatibility by trial) ANOVA was conducted. Significant main effects were found for both S-R compatibility, $F(1,1490)=227.410$, $p<0.001$, partial $\eta^2=0.132$ and for trial, $F(4,1490)=20.957$, $p<0.001$, partial $\eta^2=0.053$ (Appendix J). Higher AI scores were found for the S-R compatible condition across all subjects and assessments (Figure 12). Pairwise comparisons for trial indicated that trial 1 was significantly different than the other 4 trials ($p<0.05$, adjusted for multiple comparisons) (Figure 13).

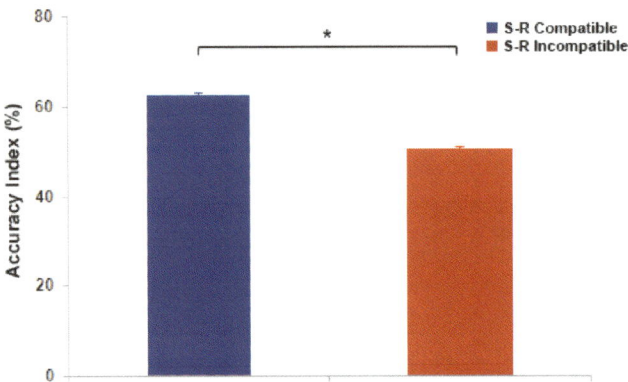

Figure 12. **Tracking accuracy (Mean ± SE) for each S-R compatibility**. Across both training groups and all assessments, higher AI scores were observed for the compatible condition compared to incompatible (* $p<0.001$).

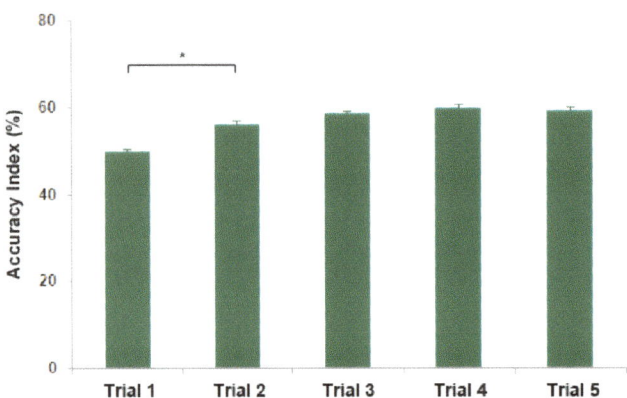

Figure 13. **Tracking accuracy (Mean ± SE) across trials**. Across both groups, all assessments and both S-R compatibility conditions, AI scores for trial 1 were lower than the other four trials (*$p<0.05$).

Significant interactions were found for S-R compatibility by assessment, $F(3,1490)=9.345$, $p<0.001$, trial by assessment, $F(12,1490)=8.208$, $p<0.001$ and, trial by S-R compatibility, $F(4,1490)=5.131$, $p<0.001$. Simple effects analyses indicated S-R compatible AI was significantly higher at post-training, 12hr and 24hr follow-up compared to pre-training. Scores were also higher at 24hr follow-up compared with post-training. S-R incompatible AI was significantly higher for all assessments compared to pre-training AI. Also, scores were higher at both follow-up assessments compared to post-training but not significantly different from one another (p<0.05, adjusted for multiple comparisons).

For the trial by assessment interaction, simple effects analyses indicated that trial 1 AI was lower than all other trials at pre-training. At 12hr follow-up, trial 1 AI scores were lower than trials 3-5 (Figure 14). No differences between trials were noted at post-training or 24hr follow-up. Across all assessments, differences in AI scores between trials was significantly affected by S-R compatibility with S-R incompatible AI scores significantly lower for the 1st and 2nd trial within an assessment while only trial 1 was found to be significantly lower for the S-R compatible condition(p<0.05, adjusted for multiple comparisons).

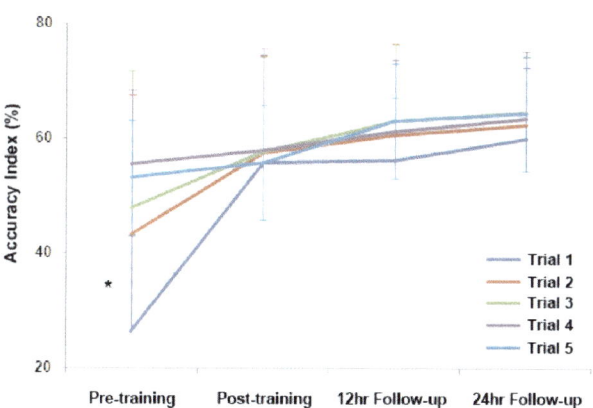

Figure 14. **Trial by assessment interaction for AI scores (Mean ± SE)**. At pre-training, AI scores for trial 1 were significantly lower than the other four trials. Trial 1 AI scores were also lower than trials 3-5 at 12hr follow-up assessment (*p<0.05).

It was assumed that trials 2-5 were a more stable and accurate assessment of level of performance, thus repeated-measures ANOVA was conducted for mean AI across trials 2-5. Trial 1 was analyzed separately for each S-R compatibility condition. Mauchly's test indicated that the assumption of sphericity was violated for the main effect of assessment; therefore, Greenhouse-Geisser adjustments were made. Results demonstrated a significant main effect of assessment for S-R compatible AI, $F(2.139, 74.877)=30.916$, $p<0.001$, partial $\eta^2=0.469$. Pairwise comparisons indicated that pre-training AI was lower than for all other assessments. Also, AI scores at both follow-up assessments were higher compared to post-training (Figure 15). A group by assessment interaction effect was not observed, $F(2.139, 74.877)$, $p=0.654$. Also, there was not a significant between-group main effect of training group, $F(1,35)=0.134$, $p=0.716$ (Appendix N).

For the S-R incompatible condition, Mauchly's test of sphericity was again significant. Results indicated a significant effect of assessment, $F(3,84.877)=28.206$, $p<0.001$, partial $\eta^2=0.446$. Accuracy was higher after training and AI was higher at both follow-up assessments compared to pre- or post-training (Figure 15). The group by assessment interaction was not significant, $F(3,84.877)=0.117$, $p=0.921$ (Appendix O).

For assessment of Trial 1 only, RM ANOVAs again revealed a significant main effect of assessment for both S-R compatibility conditions: compatible, $F(1.652,57.828)=30.326$, $p<0.001$, partial $\eta^2=0.811$, incompatible: $F(1.906,66.698)=51.678$, $p<0.001$, partial $\eta^2=0.812$. For both compatibility conditions, pre-training AI scores were lower than the other three assessments. The S-R incompatible condition demonstrated improved AI at each assessment compared to the preceding assessment while the S-R compatible condition, the two follow-up assessments did not differ significantly from post-training scores (Figure 15)(Appendices P,Q).

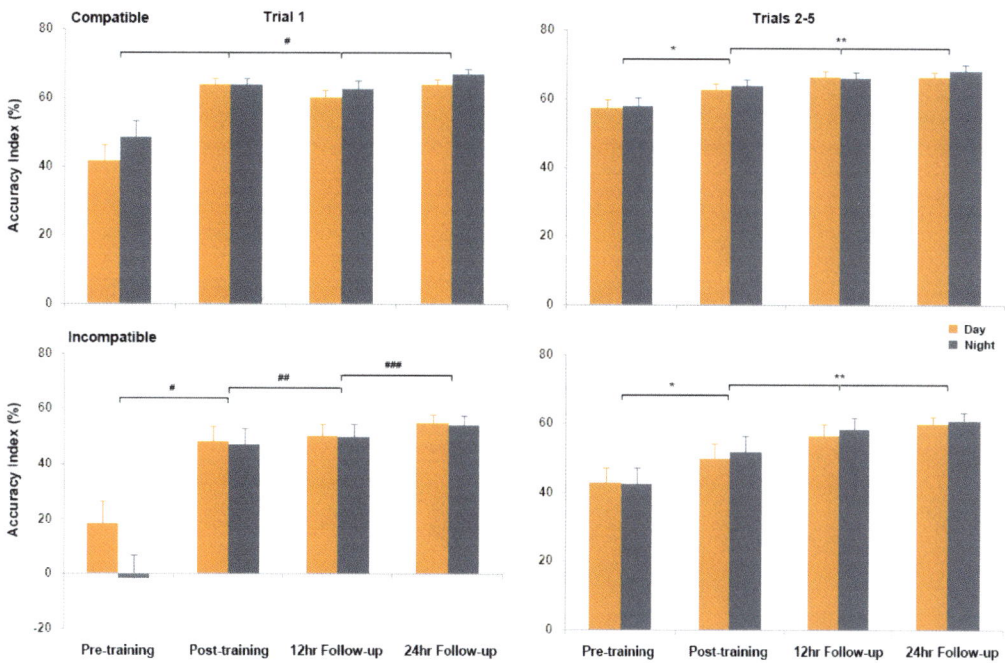

Figure 15. **Accuracy index (AI) (Mean ± SE) results between groups, across sessions, separated by S-R compatibility and trial**. Upper left panel: Trial 1 AI scores were higher at post-training, 12hr and 24hr follow-up compared to pre-training scores (#, p<0.001). Upper right panel: AI scores were higher at both follow-up assessments compared to post-training for S-R compatible trials 2-5 (**, p<0.05). Lower left panel: S-R incompatible scores were significant higher at each assessment point compared with previous assessment (#-###) p<0.05). Lower right panel: AI scores were higher at both follow-up assessments compared to post-training for S-R incompatible trials 2-5 (**, p<0.05). There were no differences between Day and Night groups.

Within-subject changes in performance were qualitatively explored to examine intra-individual differences that were not observed in group data and statistics (Appendix R).

    a. *Lag*

Normality tests for tracking lag data found violations of normality that were not amenable to data transformation processes secondary to a large percentage of cases with zero values. Parametric analyses were performed based on the robustness of RM ANOVAs. To evaluate the main effects of stimulus-response (S-R) compatibility and trial on lag, a univariate four-way ANOVA was conducted. Tests demonstrated a main effect of trial, $F(4,1490)=2.584$, $p=0.036$, partial $\eta^2=0.007$ and S-R compatibility,

F(1,1490)=50.196, p<0.001, partial η^2=0.031. Interaction effects were observed for: assessment by trial, F(12,1490)=2.406, p=0.048, partial η^2=0.021; assessment by S-R compatibility, F(3,1490)=13.258, p<0.001, partial η^2=0.026; and trial by S-R compatibility, F(4,1490)=3.905, p=0.004, partial η^2=0.010.

Simple effects analyses for significant interactions demonstrated tracking lag was different for all pairwise comparisons of trial at pre-training except between trials 2 and 3 and between 1 and 3 with decreases in lag demonstrated as trial number increased. No differences between trials were noted at any of the other three assessments. Pairwise analysis demonstrated that S-R incompatible lag was lower for all assessments when compared to pre-training and lag was reduced at 24hr follow-up compared to post-training. No differences in S-R compatible lag were observed between sessions. An effect of trial was not observed for S-R compatible condition but trial 1 was significantly lower than trials 2-5 for the S-R incompatible condition. Based on these results and the results for AI, RM ANOVAs were conducted separately for S-R compatibility conditions and for trial 1 versus trials 2-5 for the S-R incompatible condition while all 5 trials were averaged for the S-R compatible condition.

No significant main or interaction effects were observed for effects of group and assessment for S-R compatible lag. When trial 1 was examined for S-R incompatible lag, RM ANOVA demonstrated a significant main effect of assessment, F(1.910,66.867)=9.351, p<0.001, partial η^2=0.211, with higher lag values at pre-training assessment compared to the next three assessments (Appendix S). For trials 2-5, RM ANOVA again demonstrated a significant effect of assessment, F(1.805,63.160)=6.493, p=0.004, partial η^2=0.156 (Appendix T). Pairwise comparisons found pre-training lag values were larger than for each follow-up assessment but not the post-training assessment (Figure 16).

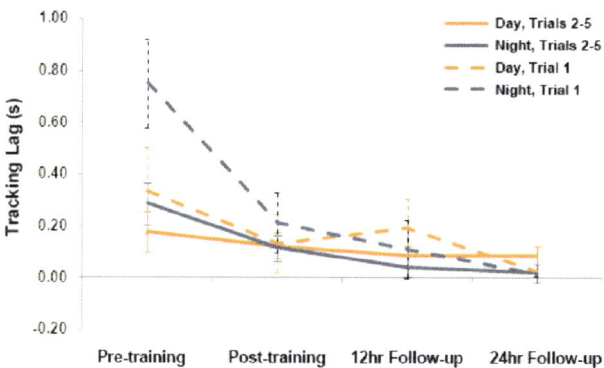

Figure 16. **Tracking lag (Mean ± SE) across sessions between groups**. No difference between groups was observed. Larger lag values were observed at pre-training assessment compared to the follow-up assessments but only trial 1 demonstrated reduced tracking lag immediately following training (p<0.05).

2. *Measurements of finger-tracking performance during the training period*

To examine for improvement that occurred within the training session, performance probes during the first and last training block were made. These data were found to be normally distributed with homogeneity of variance not violated for AI but lag data was not normally distributed with a skewed and leptokurtic shape. Data was resistant to transformation due to large number of zero values.

Repeated measures ANOVA detected a significant main effect of training block for AI, $F(1,37)=161.826$, $p<0.001$, partial $\eta^2=0.814$, with a non-significant effect of group and the interaction effect between training block and group was also not significant (Figure 17).

Repeated measures ANOVA found a significant main effect of training block for lag, $F(1,37)=16.926$, $p<0.001$, partial $\eta^2=0.314$. No effect was observed for group or the interaction effect between group and training block (Figure 17) (Appendix U).

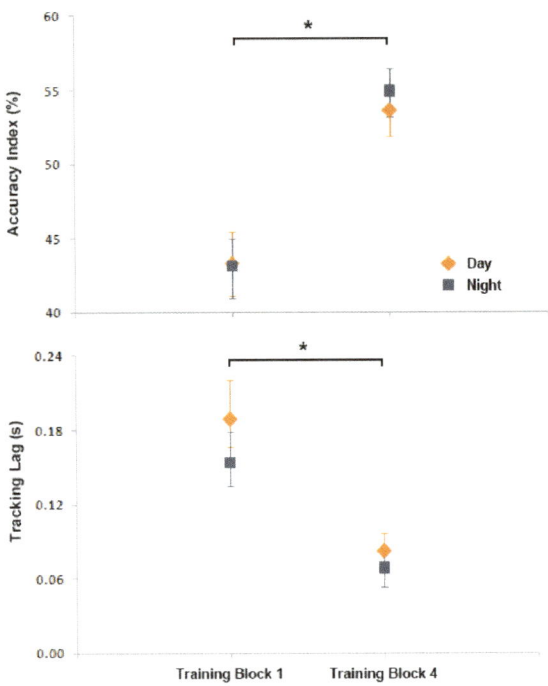

Figure 17. **Accuracy and lag values (Mean ± SE) between groups and training blocks**. Accuracy improved and tracking lag was reduced during the fourth training block compared to the first block in both groups (*, p<0.001).

B. Measures of contralateral M1 cortical excitability

1. *Single-pulse (SP) MEP amplitude*

Data were found to significantly violate the assumptions of normality demonstrated by a negatively skewed (skewness=1.616) and leptokurtic (kurtosis=2.731) distribution. Following log transform, the data were found assume a normal distribution, therefore, parametric analyses were conducted (Appendix V).

To evaluate the potential effect of SP test order (either pre-PP or post-PP), a three-way (group x assessment x test order) univariate ANOVA revealed a significant interaction effect for group by assessment, $F(3,3107)=3.361$, $p=0.018$, and for group by test order, $F(1,3251)=12.344$, $p<0.001$. Small effect sizes were found for both results (partial η^2=0.003, 0.004). Simple effects analyses indicated a significant change in SP MEP from pre-training to post-training in the Day training group and from post-training to 24hr follow-up. No differences were observed within the Night training group. Another three-way ANOVA was conducted with group, assessment and trial as factors. A main effect of trial was not observed but a significant interaction effect was found for group by trial, $F(19,3107)=1.651$, $p=0.037$. Again, the effect size was small for this term, partial $\eta^2=0.010$. Simple effects analyses demonstrated a significant effect of trial within the Day group with no significant effect observed for the Night group (Appendix W).

Collapsed across trial, repeated-measures ANOVAs did not detect significant main effects for assessment or group, nor was an interaction effect between these terms observed (Figure 18).

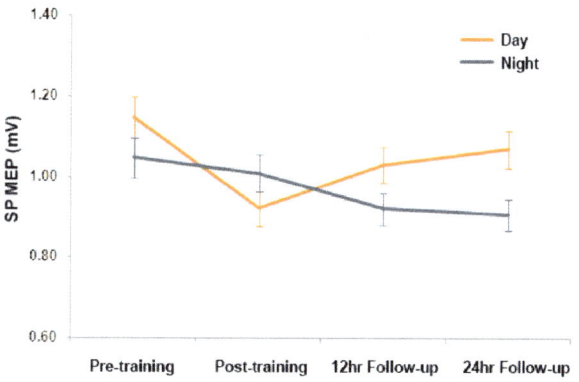

Figure 18. **SP MEP data (Mean ± SE) across assessments, between groups**. No significant differences between groups or across assessments were observed ($p>0.05$).

2. *Paired-pulse MEP ratios*

Data were found to substantially violate the assumptions of normality with a negatively skewed (skewness=2.242) and leptokurtic (kurtosis: 7.996) distribution. Log transform allowed the data to meet assumptions of normality and subsequent analyses were conducted on the transformed data (Appendix V).

Four-way (group by assessment by trial by ISI) ANOVA demonstrated significant main effects of group, $F(1,3100)=25.314$, $p<0.001$, trial, $F(9,3100)=2.434$, $p=0.009$, partial $\eta^2=0.006$, and ISI, $F(1,3100)=884.903$, $p<0.001$, partial $\eta^2=0.217$ (Figure 19). An interaction between group and ISI was found, $F(3,3120)=58.617$, $p<0.001$, partial

η^2=0.018. Pairwise comparisons demonstrated a significant trial difference between trial 1 and trial 9. Simple effects analyses identified significant group differences at each ISI, with a larger mean difference for ISI=3ms (SICI), 0.220, compared to ISI=10ms (ICF), 0.009 (Appendix X). Subsequent RM ANOVAs were conducted on mean log-transformed PP ratio data separately for each ISI (3ms,10ms). For ISI=3ms, a trend for a main effect of group was observed, $F(1,36)$=3.861, $p<0.057$. Main effects of group and assessment were not found for ISI=10ms. An interaction between the main effects was also not observed for either ISI (Appendix Y).

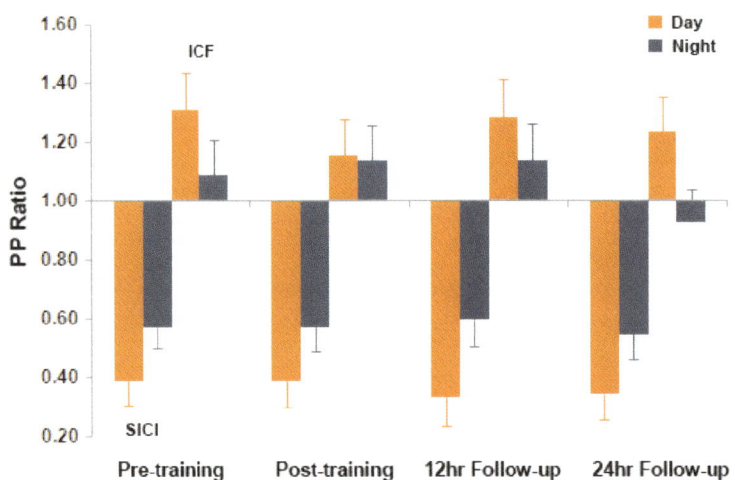

Figure 19. **PP ratios across assessments, between groups (Mean ± SE)**. Values indicated a short ISI (3ms) reduced test pulse MEP while a longer ISI (10ms) increased the test pulse MEP ($p<0.001$).

3. *CSP*

Data were normally distributed for CSP across all subjects. The assumption of homogeneity of variance was not violated.

A three-way ANOVA (group x assessment x trial) did not demonstrate a significant main effect of trial, $F(9,1534)$=0.349, p=0.958, or interaction effects of trial with group, $F(9,1534)$=0.107, p=1.00, or assessment, $F(27,1534)$=0.181, p=1.00. Therefore, subsequent RM ANOVAs were conducted on mean CSP data. No significant main

(F(2.542,88.972)=0.700, p=0.532) or interaction effects (F(2.542,88.972)=0.631, p=0.571) were found for group or assessment for mean CSP.

4. *TMS-evoked motor thresholds*

Data were normally distributed for each threshold (rMT, aMT, 1mVT). Homogeneity of variance was confirmed. For each threshold, repeated-measures ANOVA were conducted.

   a. *Resting motor threshold (rMT)*

Mauchly's test indicated that the assumption of sphericity was violated for the main effect of test assessment. A significant main effect of assessment on rMT, F(2.322, 81.274)=4.955, p=0.007, partial η^2=0.124, was observed. Pairwise comparisons revealed that rMT was higher following training compared with other assessments (Figure 20). There was also a trend for an interaction effect observed between assessment and group, F(2.322, 81.274)=2.857, p=0.055, partial η^2=0.075, where rMT was higher in the Day training group at post-training. Multivariate tests did demonstrate a significant interaction effect for this term, Wilks' λ=0.781, F(3,33)=3.085, p=0.041, partial η^2=0.219. The between-subjects effect of group was not significant, F(1,35)=1.337, p=0.255 (Appendix Z).

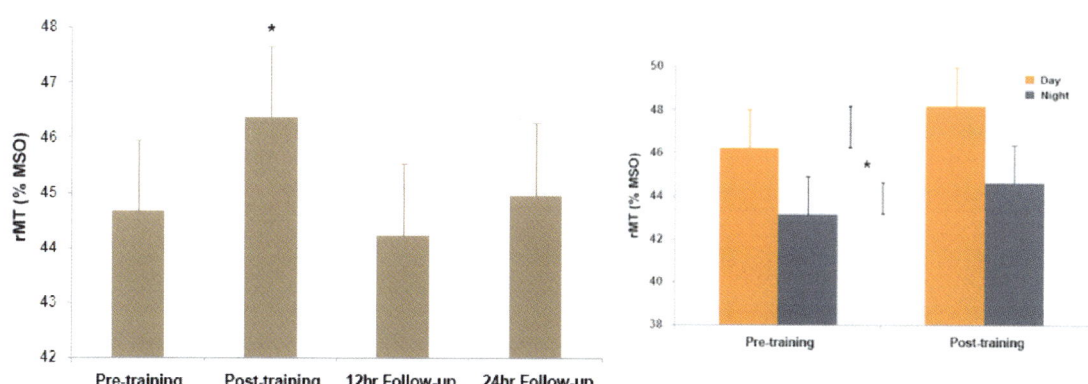

Figure 20. **Resting motor threshold (rMT) across sessions (Mean ± SE).** Left) Increased rMT observed following training across all subjects (*, p<0.05). Right) This change was greater in the Day training group (*, p<0.05).

b. Active motor threshold (aMT)

A significant between-subjects effect of group was observed, $F(1,35)=4.852$, $p=0.034$, partial $\eta^2=0.122$, where subjects in the Day training group had higher aMT values across assessments (Figure 21) (Appendix AA).

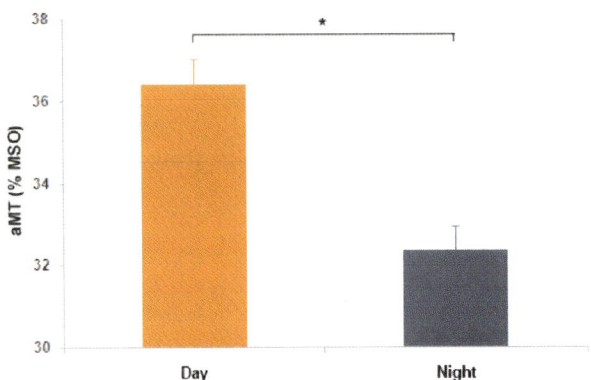

Figure 21. **Active motor threshold (aMT) values between groups (Mean ± SE)**. Across all assessment, aMT values were higher in the day training group (*, $p<0.05$).

c. 1mV threshold (1mVT)

The group by assessment interaction term was found to be significant using multivariate tests, Wilks' $\lambda=0.781$, $F(3,33)=2.977$, $p=0.046$, partial $\eta^2=0.213$. A trend for a within-subjects interaction was observed, $F(3,105)=2.391$, $p=0.073$, partial $\eta^2=0.064$ (Figure 22) (Appendix BB).

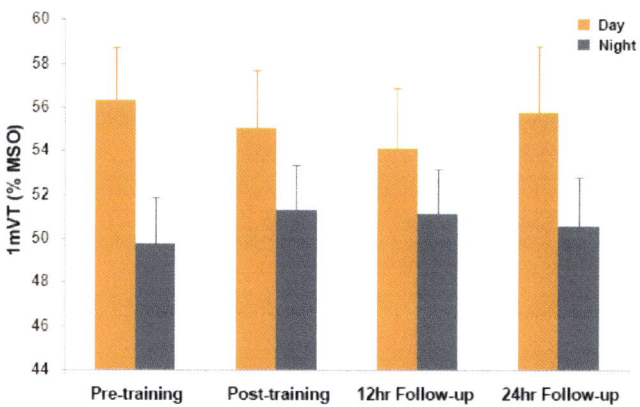

Figure 22. **One millivolt threshold (1mVT) values across assessments (Mean ± SE).** Between groups, there was a trend for a group by assessment interaction (p=0.073) with increased 1mVT from pre-training to post-training/12hr follow-up in the night group, while there was a trend for decreased 1mVT in the day group from pre-training to post-training/12hr follow-up.

C. Actigraphic assessment of sleep

Measures of sleep quality (Sleep efficiency, Time asleep, Time awake, Awakenings, Average Time Awake, Sleep Latency), did not substantially violate the assumptions of normality and homogeneity of variance. All measures of sleep quality were significantly (p<0.05) correlated to one another across both nights of sleep (Pearson's r range: .230-.925) (Appendix CC). These measures were also correlated with subjective report of sleep quality (PSQI) and sleepiness (ESS).

Multivariate ANOVA did not demonstrate significant main effects for training group, $F(6,64)=1.4.66$, p=0.204, or night of sleep (before training or the night following training), $F(6,64)=0.884$, p=0.512, nor was an interaction effect between these terms observed, $F(6,64)=0.744$, p=0.616.

D. Relationship between tracking performance and subject characteristics

AI and Gender were correlated at pre-training assessment, Pearson's r=-0.577, with females exhibiting lower AI scores before training. Hierarchical regression demonstrated that gender was a significant predictor of AI, $R^2=0.333$, β=-0.159. Casewise diagnostics identified one extreme outlier in the data set (>3SD). When removed, the correlation between gender and AI increased, Pearson's r=-0.616 and the predictive capacity of the model improved, R^2=0.380, β=-0.139. Adding age to the model did not significantly improve the model (Appendix DD). At 12hr follow-up assessment, across both skill training groups, gender was correlated with change in AI from post-training assessment, Pearson's r=0.383 and was a significant predictor of change in AI, R^2=0.147, β=0.044, indicating females had higher AI change scores following the first post-training interval (Appendix EE).

E. *Relationship between tracking performance and cortical excitability*

AI was not significantly related to SP or PP measures of CE at pre-training. At 12hr follow-up, PP measures (SICI and ICF) of excitability were correlated with AI, r=-.347,-.383, and predictive of AI, R^2=0.235, βs=-0.072, -0.145 (Appendix FF). Casewise diagnostics identified two extreme outliers in the data set. When removed, the correlation between AI and measures of PP was stronger, r=-0.504, -0.536 and, the predictive capacity of the model improved, R^2=0.476, β=-0.075, =0.145 (Figure 23). When examining the Day training group at 12hr follow-up, SICI remained correlated with AI, r=-.419 but ICF was no longer significantly related to AI. The regression model was also not significant for SICI and ICF. In the Night training group, SICI was not significantly associated with AI, r=-.344 but ICF was correlated with AI, r=-.647. The regression model exhibited significant predictive value of SICI and ICF for AI, R^2=0.451, βs=-0.034, -0.169. At 24hr assessment, PP measures were not predictive of tracking accuracy variance in either group (Appendix GG).

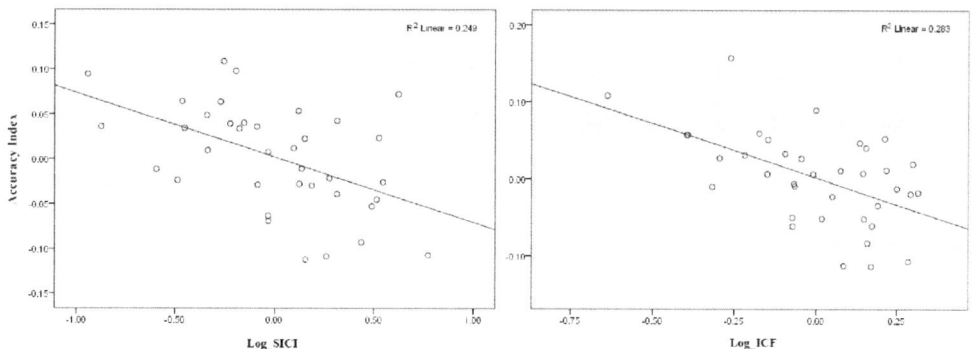

Figure 23. **Partial regression plots for relationship between tracking performance and paired-pulse MEP ratios at 12hr follow-up in both groups.** Tracking performance was associated with intracortical excitability where increased accuracy was predicted by decreased excitability (p<0.001).

Tracking performance was not correlated with CSP at any assessment for either group. At pre-training assessment, AI was positively correlated with rMT, r=0.253, p<0.05, but not with aMT or 1mVT. As the sole predictor, rMT was not a significant predictor of the variance in AI, R^2=0.064, βs=0.253, p=0.083. When 1mVT was added in the model, the model reached significance, R^2=0.156, βs=-0.654, -0.503, p=0.022. The addition of aMT did not improve the predictive capacity of the model. This relationship was also observed for both S-R compatibility conditions: compatible: R^2=0.138, βs=0.611, -0.530, p=0.036, incompatible: R^2=0.136, βs=0.605, -0.431, p=0.038 (Appendix HH). A significant relationship was not observed between thresholds and AI immediately following training.

F. Relationship between tracking performance and sleep characteristics

Measures of sleep quality did not significantly predict variance in AI at pre-training, regardless of S-R compatibility. At 12hr follow-up, the preceding night's sleep quality (Night 1 for Day training and Night 2 for Night training) was a significant predictor of AI with differential effects for compatibility between groups. For the day group, there was a trend for sleep quality as a predictor of the variance in S-R compatible AI, R^2=0.300, βs=-0.547, -0.470, p=0.059 (Appendix II) (Figure 24), while sleep quality in the Night group was predictive of the variance in S-R incompatible AI, R^2=0.333, βs=0.349, 0.620 p=0.048 (Appendix JJ) (Figure 25). This relationship was maintained at 24hr follow-up,

R^2=0.363, βs=0.582, 0.583, p=0.043 (Appendix KK). Sleep quality was not predictive of the change in AI from post-training to 12hr follow-up in either group. Night 2 sleep quality was a significant predictor of the change in S-R compatible AI from post-training assessment to 24hr follow-up in the Day group, R^2=0.644, βs=-0.411, 0.195, 0.829, p<0.001 (Appendix LL) (Figure 26).

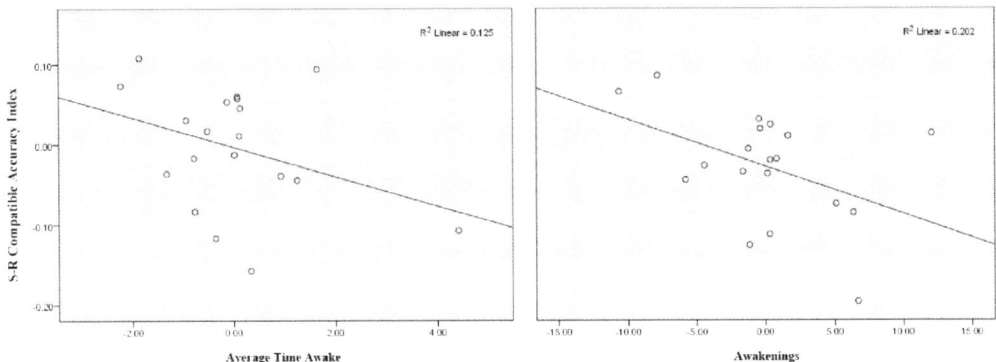

Figure 24. **Partial regression plots for relationship between tracking performance and sleep quality at 12hr follow-up in the Day group.** A trend was observed for a predictive relationship for preceding night sleep quality and subsequent tracking following training (p=0.057).

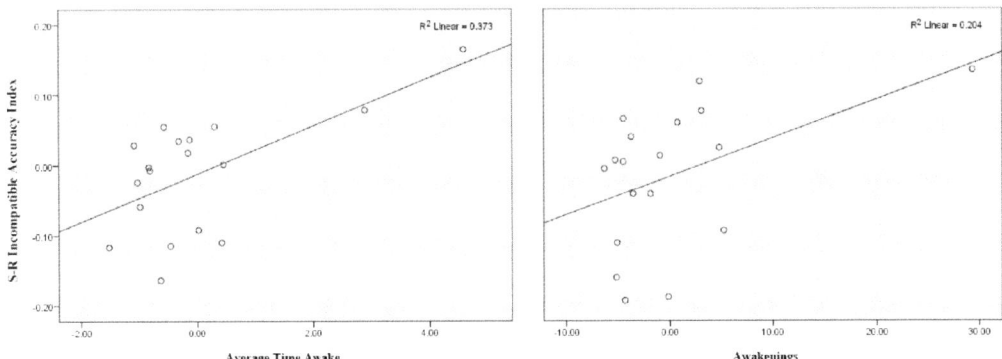

Figure 25. **Partial regression plots for relationship between tracking performance and sleep quality at 12hr follow-up in the Night group.** A predictive relationship for preceding night sleep quality and subsequent tracking following training was observed (p=0.048).

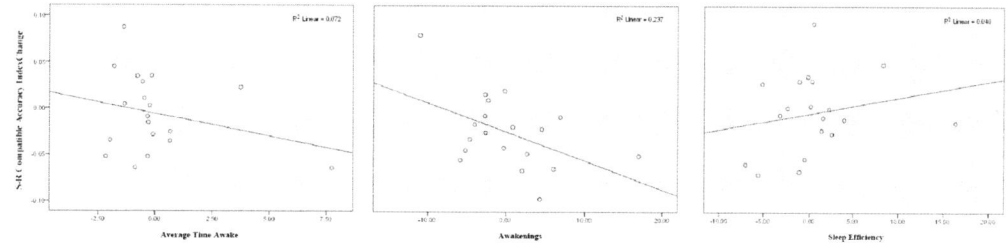

Figure 26. **Partial regression plots for relationship between change in tracking performance and sleep quality at 24hr follow-up in the Day group.** A predictive relationship for preceding night sleep quality and change in tracking performance from post-training to 24hr follow-up was observed (p=0.001).

G. *Effect of skilled tracking training versus repeated, simple movement*

1. *Subject characteristics*

No differences (p>0.05) were observed between skill training and movement groups for age, gender, handedness or subjective sleep quality or sleepiness (Table 4).

Table 4: Demographic data

Group	Age	Gender	EHI	PSQI	ESS	SSS (pre)	SSS (post)	SSS (12hr)	SSS (24hr)
Skill	22.6 ± 3.9	M:20, F:20	76.1 ± 21.2	4.3 ± 2.1	7.3 ± 3.6	2.5 ± 1.0	2.5 ± 1.2	2.3 ± 1.2	2.3 ± 0.9
Move	23.8 ± 2.0	M:5, F:5	88.1 ± 25.2	4.6 ± 2.2	7.4 ± 1.3	2.2 ± 0.9	2.4 ± 1.0	2.4 ± 0.5	2.1 ± 1.0

EHI: Edinburgh Handedness Inventory; PSQI: Pittsburgh Sleep Quality Index; ESS: Epworth Sleepiness Scale; SSS: Stanford Sleepiness Scale

2. *Tracking performance*

No significant differences in tracking performance following skill training versus repeated, simple movement were observed for either S-R compatibility condition (Trials 2-5: compatible: p=0.263, incompatible: p=0.917) (Figure 23). No difference was observed for all trials (compatible: p=0.167, incompatible: p=0.908) or when only trial 1 was analyzed (compatible: p=0.126, incompatible: p=0.812) (Appendix MM).

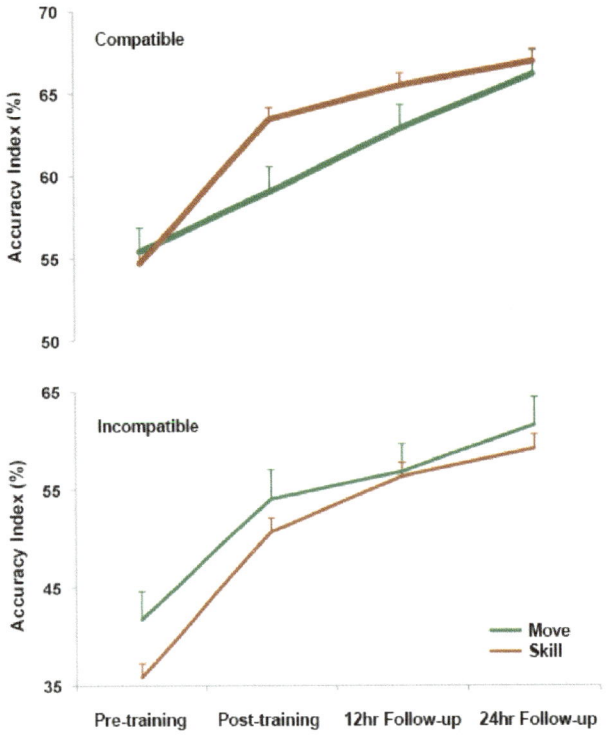

Figure 27. **Tracking performance (Mean ± SE, trials 2-5) across assessments between skill training and movement activity.** No significant differences were found between groups for tracking accuracy for either compatibility condition across assessments.

3. *Cortical excitability*

Repeated measures ANOVA did not determine a significant effect of training versus simple movement on measures of cortical excitability at any assessment. No significant differences in thresholds were observed between training and move groups ($p>0.05$).

4. *Sleep quality*

There were no differences in sleep quality for between training and the move groups found for either night ($p>0.05$).

H. Null hypotheses decisions

H1$_o$. Motor skill training **would not** improve immediate skill performance.

a$_o$. Following motor skill training, skill performance at P2 **would not** be improved compared to P1. **Reject**

b$_o$. Improvement **would** be affected by time of training. **Reject**

H2$_o$. Skill development **would not** be dependent on first post-training interval

a$_o$. Following a waking interval, there **would not** be significant skill improvement in the Day training group at F1. **Reject**

b$_o$. Following an interval containing sleep, there **would not** be significant motor learning improvement in the Night training group at F1. **Reject**

c$_o$. These changes (H2a. and H2b.) **would not** be affected by time of training evidenced by no change in performance improvement at F1 when the first post-training interval contains sleep compared to waking activity. **Fail to reject**

d$_o$. Within training groups, skill performance at F2 **would** be different than at F1. **Reject**

e$_o$. Skill performance at F2 **would not** remain higher in the Night training group compared to performance in the Day group. **Fail to reject**

H3$_o$. Cortical excitability (CE) **would not** be increased following skill training.

a$_o$. Measures of CE (single-pulse MEP, paired pulse MEP, CSP duration and TMS-evoked thresholds) **would not** demonstrate significantly increased primary motor cortex excitability at P2, after finger-tracking training, compared to P1. **Fail to reject**

b$_o$. Measures of CE **would not** be significantly reduced at both post-training intervals (F1, F2) compared to post-training results, but would not be significantly different from CE at P1. **Fail to reject**

c$_o$. Increases in CE following training **would** be dependent on time of training. **Reject**

H4$_o$. Sleep quality and sleepiness **would** be different across groups or testing sessions.

a_o. There **would** be a difference in sleep quality across groups for either night of sleep (N1 or N2). **Reject**

b_o. Preceding night sleep quality **would not** be positively associated with skill performance at P1 and F1 for Night group and F2 for Day group. **Reject**

c_o. The relationship between sleep quality and tracking performance between training groups **would** be different at for least one assessment. **Fail to reject**

$H5_o$. Motor skill training **would not** enhance skill performance in the training group compared to the movement group.

a_o. Motor skill training **would not** significantly improve finger-tracking accuracy at P2 compared to unskilled, repeated finger movement. **Fail to reject**

b_o. Finger-tracking accuracy **would not** be significantly greater for the training groups than observed for the movement group at both F1 and F2. **Fail to reject**

I. Retrospective power analyses of results for primary H_os

$H2c_o$: Mean AI difference between groups (Night-Day) for change (12hr follow-up-post-training) in mean AI (both compatibility conditions) =-0.5, σ_{Day}= 11.5, σ_{Night}=11.5, n=20, n=20. Required sample size: **n=2226/sample**. S-R compatible AI change difference=-0.8, σ_{Day}= 8.5, σ_{Night}=8.5, n=20, n=20. Required sample size: **n=460/sample**. S-R incompatible AI change difference=-2.6, σ_{Day}= 11.7, σ_{Night}=22.6, n=20, n=20. Required sample size: **n=32053/sample**.

$H3a_o$: Mean (all trials) PP ratio (log-transformed) (ISI=3ms) difference between pre- and post-training assessments=-0.05, σ_{pre}= 0.23, σ_{post}=0.29, n=38, n=38. Required sample size: **n=320/sample**. PP ratio (ISI=10ms) difference=-0.001, σ_{pre}= 0.21, σ_{post}=0.17, n=38, n=38. Required sample size: **n=333731**/sample.

$H5a_o$: Mean (all trials) S-R compatible AI difference between skill and move groups (post-training-pre-training) =5.1, σ_{Skill}=8.9 σ_{Move}=8.9, n=37, n=9. Required sample size: **n=15/sample**. Mean (all trials) S-R incompatible AI difference=2.3, σ_{Skill}=29.3, σ_{Move}=31.1, n=37, n=9. Required sample size: **n=836/sample**.

V. Discussion

A. *Summary of major findings*

The role of sleep on memory formation remains predominately unknown. Previous research has provided data to support sleep-dependent memory consolidation processes can result in offline skill enhancement following exposure to certain motor skills. This investigation has attempted to contribute to this area of research by investigating the effect of different post-training intervals; one interval only involving waking activity and one interval containing sleep, on the offline development of a novel, goal-directed visuospatial motor skill.

The primary results of this work support previous literature indicating that motor skills can continue to develop following training but did not confirm the primary hypothesis that sleep following training would confer additional benefits to this observed offline skill enhancement. A second major finding was that measures of cortical excitability were modified by skill training, but were not influenced by the time of day. Thirdly, objective sleep quality following training was predictive of the level of skill performance in the next follow-up skill assessment and a differential effect of task complexity was observed between training groups. Lastly, when comparing skilled finger-tracking training to an equivalent period of repeated, unskilled finger movement, no significant differences in skill development were found between these two groups. Here, each major finding will be enumerated and discussed in light of the observed results and within the context of previous literature, current study limitations and future research applications.

1. **Finger tracking skill performance improved following training and improvement was not only retained after 12- and 24-hr intervals but was enhanced compared to post-training level of skill. This enhancement was not significantly increased by an interval containing sleep versus an interval containing only waking activity.**

Finger-tracking performance, represented by accuracy index (AI) and lag scores, significantly improved immediately following one twenty-minute training period designed to promote skill development in both the day and night training groups. These findings indicate that time of day did not significantly affect initial skill acquisition or immediate performance. This improvement in skill performance demonstrates that rapid skill acquisition occurred for this goal-directed, visuospatial finger-tracking skill. These data are also in line with previous results for a similar training paradigm[53].

In an effort to control for practice effects that may have been associated with repeated trials of the same waveform, within-assessment analyses were conducted to evaluate trial-by-trial tracking performance. As expected, during pre-training skill assessment, there was a significant improvement from the first trial to the next four trials for each S-R compatibility condition. Importantly, this assessment was the only assessment where a trial effect was observed. This suggests that between-session skill enhancement was not due to practice-dependent improvement within a given assessment but, rather, retention of previously acquired information over time. The lack of within-assessment differences between trials immediately following training supports that asymptotic performance occurred and the lack of a trial effect at either follow-up session argues against significant improvements in tracking skill performance due to repeated exposures to the test waveform. These results argue that the majority of skill acquisition took place during the training assessment and between-session skill retention occurred for the acquired information.

Sleep has been shown to benefit learning for a number of motor skills[7, 77, 79] but the results of this experiment did not indicate a substantive benefit of sleep following training compared to an equivalent period of waking activity. It was hypothesized that the skill employed here would preferentially benefit from sleep following training due to the complexity of the task. This task required continuous visuospatial processing to accurately track a computer-generated waveform using the dominant index finger. Subjects were also given visual feedback of real-time performance; therefore, online movement control in response to visual information was required. Lastly, all subjects had explicit awareness of the goal of the task: track the computer-generated waveform as accurately as possible for the entire duration of the trial. In designing the components of the task, it was argued that the dynamic, continuous nature of the task, combined with visuomotor processing demands and cognitive awareness of the goal of the task, would produce a more complex motor skill to be learned than skills learning in previous experiments. However, this may not be the case. Although the tracking apparatus is novel, controlled movements of the dominant index finger with on-line movement correction occurs repeatedly during daily skills. This does make the selected motor task an attractive tool to assess and improve functional hand control in patient populations[128, 143], but it may lack the required complexity to challenge a healthy neuromuscular system. Supporting this speculation are the rapid improvements in tracking performance observed within the first skill assessment. As discussed previously, sleep has been shown to benefit tasks that are more complex[11, 39, 57] while the mere passage of time provides greater benefit simple movement skills[57, 58].

Another factor to consider is that the chosen measurements of tracking performance do not probe the specific parameters of motor control patterns that may have been preferentially modified by sleep. However, the accuracy index has previously been shown to be a reliable and valid measure of motor skill performance and assessment of skill improvement over time[52, 128, 144] making this a relatively unlikely mechanism for the observed results. Given the results of this study, we feel the most likely factor for lack of effect is that visuomotor skill learning does not require sleep-dependent memory consolidation processes observed for other motor skills and the simple passage of time is sufficient for offline skill enhancement to occur. A number of recent studies have shown that certain skills, in fact, do not benefit from sleep following skill acquisition.

Previous work demonstrating a beneficial effect of sleep in post-training skill enhancement has primarily utilized serial reaction finger tapping sequence learning[11, 43, 60] where the skill is acquired without conscious awareness. This is achieved by embedding a repeated sequence during a training period of random sequence tapping. Skill is measured by the difference in reaction time between repeated and random sequences during the training session and typically after a 12hr interval containing either sleep or no sleep. This task can also be presented explicitly where subjects spend a training period performing the same four-element tapping sequence as quickly and accurately as possible[39, 44]. Reaction time and number of repeated sequences completed correctly are usual indicators of performance. In both task paradigms, robust enhancement of skill performance in terms of reaction time, but not accuracy, is observed after a night of sleep. Results also suggest that explicit awareness of the task and increased complexity of the task benefit from sleep to a greater extent than simple, implicit sequence learning [11, 39, 57].

As discussed in the introduction, sequential tapping motor skill learning has limited "real life" application to (re)learning of functional skills. The main transferrable component is the discrete nature of the task since many functional skills are multi-step processes. Yet, these multi-step processes are usually learned with explicit awareness of the goal of the task and the accuracy of the movement produced. Also, the multi-step nature of functional tasks typically occurs over a different time span compared to repeatedly tapping four fingers in sequence as quickly as possible. Finger-sequence learning also differs from most functional skills in terms of the perceptual demands required for successful performance. Finger tapping uses a visual cue presented sequentially to prompt a key press but rarely is feedback provided to allow for online performance adjustment. Therefore, minimal feedforward or feedback processing is required to complete the task successfully. As a result, it is likely that this skill uses different motor control programs based on the time constraints and information used to produce skilled movement compared functional motor skills[14].

Relatedly, reaction time as a measure of skill proficiency has limited application to functional task performance. Skills are rarely performed with speed of movement as the goal. Far more often, the quality or accuracy of the movement is what is meaningful. The differences between discrete finger-tapping sequence learning and the task employed here are substantial enough to explain the apparent discrepancy in the beneficial role for sleep in offline memory enhancement. Other motor learning paradigms also argue for the conclusion supported by these data: sleep-dependent motor skill memory enhancement is contingent on the nature of the skill to be learned.

Another factor to consider in sleep and motor skill learning paradigms is the effect of circadian rhythms and time of day of training and/or skill assessment. Recent investigations have begun to separate these effects by training subjects and assessing skill performance at different times of day. Keisler and colleagues[145] showed that skill performance improvements overnight were not significantly greater than improvements observed for a group that had the same amount of skill practice but did not sleep between assessments. These data illustrate the limitation of assessing skill performance only before and after sleep since the overnight improvements observed may just be a recovery of skill performance, not an actual indicator of skill learning. The authors argue that the results indicate that the systematic variance in time of day creates a significant confound in typical sleep and learning studies. A similar training paradigm corroborated[146] these findings and contrasted previous work indicating a significant role for sleep in the offline consolidation of sequence skill learning[7, 12, 43].

Our work has attempted to control for this potential confounding effect by assessing performance of all subjects after an interval with and without sleep after training has occurred. Our findings suggest that sleep did not simply reverse the negative time of day effect of skill performance assessment in the evening immediately following training since subjects trained during the day also demonstrated similar performance improvement over a day of waking activity. Additionally, improvements at 12hr follow-up, regardless of time of assessment, were maintained at 24hr follow-up. Therefore, the study design employed demonstrated offline skill enhancement that could not be explained by factors associated with time of day such as fatigue, motivation or attention[147].

The influence of sleep on motor skill learning has been examined using two other types of motor skills that are continuous in nature: dynamic visuomotor adaptation and implicit visuospatial tracking. In adaptation learning, subjects learn to accurately produce a 'target-out' reaching movement using a manipulandum or joystick[44, 148]. This movement can occur over multiple joint segments depending on the distance between the starting position and target and the apparatus used[44, 59]. It can be learned with a perturbation by a velocity-dependent force field applied perpendicular to the movement[59] or by training on an inverted condition (S-R incompatible) where visual feedback of the movement produced is in the opposite direction of the sensory information of the movement itself[44]. In both paradigms, movement is continuous and a continuous measure of accuracy is collected, usually pathway deviation. It has been shown that in either case, offline motor skill stabilization and even enhancement occurs following training and is not dependent on sleep during this memory processing stage in young, healthy individuals[44, 149].

Another motor skill that shares many common features with the finger-tracking task employed here is implicit visuospatial tracking. This task involves continuously tracking a computer-generated target that moves in a repeated, pre-determined pattern. During tracking, the subject is able to see the target and the cursor but visual feedforward or feedback information is eliminated. Using this task, Siengsukon and Boyd[71] demonstrated the absence of offline skill enhancement in young, healthy individuals following sleep. Additionally, no increases in tracking accuracy were observed following waking. These data support previous conclusions that implicit skill learning does not benefit significantly from sleep and were extended to a continuous tracking skill. Here, the task was also a continuous tracking skill but was constrained to one joint and individuals were provided online feedforward and feedback information regarding the task and the performance of the task. The additional explicit information provided did not result in sleep-dependent offline skill enhancement, but did benefit from the passage of time following training for continued skill development.

Taken together, previous research and the results observed here argue that the beneficial effect of sleep on post-training information processing is task-dependent. It appears that continuous, explicit visuospatial finger-tracking skill development is not sensitive to post-training level of activity or arousal. These findings, combined with previous studies, suggest that sleep-dependent enhancement occurs for tasks that are discrete in nature, that do not rely on substantial perceptual processing, and where skill is evaluated by reaction time rather than accuracy over time.

2. **Neural processes underlying motor skill learning as measured by cortical excitability in the contralateral primary motor cortex were modified by skill training, but were not influenced by the time of day.**

An increase in cortical excitability (CE) was not observed following training in either training group. In fact, rMT was significantly higher across groups after training, indicating reduced cortical excitability, specifically at the neuronal membrane[106]. These data indicate that one episode of skilled finger-tracking training does not substantially modify immediate post-training excitability in the contralateral M1. This was an unexpected outcome and did not confirm our hypothesis that CE would be increased immediately following training. Previous work using various neuroimaging approaches has demonstrated involvement of M1 in skill acquisition and post-training memory consolidation[122, 150, 151]. A number of studies have shown substantial changes in cortical representations following skill training[122, 152]. These changes in activity have been shown to be specific to the trained cortical representation in M1[79, 122, 152]. Other work has demonstrated increases in M1 excitability immediately following training[122, 153]. Importantly, these effects are transient and appear to occur early during the skill acquisition phase of motor learning[21, 154, 155]. Here, significant acquisition was not accompanied by expected increases in M1 excitability. This may have been due to a number of factors.

Based on evaluation of tracking skill performance across assessments, it appears that proficiency was rapidly attained; therefore, expected increases in M1 excitability may have occurred prior to the post-training assessment over the twenty-minute training session and/or during pre-training skill assessment. Previous work has shown that once a motor skill has been learned, increases in M1 excitability are no longer observed[153, 155]. This may be due to changes in activity patterns associated with changes in skill performance.[155].

Other research has demonstrated dynamic shifts in cortical activation can occur rapidly or gradually depending on the type of motor skill trained and the relative degree to which learning has occurred over time[156]. This shift may occur across different time periods depending on the skill learned and the training paradigm[155, 156]. We previously reported that following training using the same tracking apparatus SP MEP amplitude was decreased[53]. Similar findings were observed in this investigation with increased rMT values following training indicating decreased contralateral M1 excitability. Therefore, once significant skill acquisition occurred for visuospatial finger-tracking, a shift in cortical activity from M1 to either subcortical and/or parietal associative cortices may explain the observed reduction in M1 excitability.

It appears that early motor skill performance requires substantial neural resources responsible for sensorimotor integration, motor planning, and executive functioning to accomplish a skill successfully but once learned, efficient neural processing is then associated with successful performance [42, 157]. Although dynamic changes in regional brain activity were not monitored here, it has been shown previously that regional reductions in brain activity were associated with local reductions in cortical excitability [158]. Therefore, dynamic changes in brain activity patterns from predominately cortical, prior to training, to subcortical, once the skill is learned and automated, may explain the reductions in cortical excitability after training. It may also explain the observed relationship between skill performance and intracortical M1 excitability at follow-up assessments where increased intracortical inhibition in M1 was associated with increased skill performance.

Regression analyses demonstrated a significant relationship between intracortical CE (SICI/ICF) and tracking performance at 12hr follow-up assessment. Higher SICI and lower ICF values were associated with better tracking performance. These results parallel recent findings that demonstrated reduced CE at follow-up assessment was associated with higher accuracy scores[53]. Combined, these results suggest that decreases in intracortical excitability are associated with increases in finger tracking accuracy between pre-training and 24-hour follow-up assessments. There may be multiple explanations for this finding. Contralateral M1 may be differentially recruited based on the amount and time of exposure to this skill. It has been shown using fMRI that neural activity in cortical regions, including contralateral M1, decreases following short-term visuomotor learning[155]. It appears that this shift in cortical activation can occur rapidly or gradually depending on the type of motor skill trained and the relative degree to which has been learned over time[156]. As discussed above, our results and previous research suggest a dynamic nature of brain activation patterns shifting from widely-distributed cortical activation during early performance and learning to subcortical activation once the task has been learned and largely automated. This shift may occur across different time periods depending on the skill learned and the training paradigm[155, 156].

Investigations using rTMS to produce a virtual lesion to a specific cortical region have provided results that allow for inference of causal relationships between localized brain regions and behavior that are time-dependent. As discussed in the introduction, contralateral M1 has been shown to be necessary for post-training memory consolidation for ballistic[123] and implicit sequence[60] motor skill learning, but not for dynamic adaptation[45] or explicit, continuous, visuospatial skill learning[53]. Using the same tracking apparatus, Carey and colleagues[129], demonstrated that rTMS-induced disruption of contralateral M1 did not affect initial skill acquisition but, when applied to the ipsilateral cortex, early skill acquisition was decreased. These interventional studies demonstrate that the importance of M1, both contralateral and ipsilateral to the trained extremity, for motor skill learning is dependent both on the type of skill learned and stage of information processing.

Other motor regions of the cortex, subcortical areas and the cerebellum are also engaged in the processing of motor skill information but were not objectively assessed here, nor were the relationships between brain regions assessed. It is difficult to objectively assess concurrent neural activity from different regions of the brain using a single neuroimaging technique such as TMS[159, 160]. It also has been argued that the limitations of individual neuroimaging modalities can be mitigated when combined[161]. Recent investigations have begun to incorporate multimodal imaging techniques to address the spatial and temporal limitations of these techniques when used in isolation in an effort to better elucidate neurophysiologic mechanisms underlying behavior[160, 162]. The results here demonstrate a substantial learning effect with modest changes in cortical excitability in the contralateral M1. It may be that other cortical regions were involved to a greater extent in this type of skill learning. Or, as argued above, excitability changes in M1 may have been transient and insignificant once training was completed. Future work should utilize multimodal neuroimaging approaches to simultaneously monitor multiple brain regions over the time course of skill development to better understand the interconnected relationships between motor regions of the brain at different stages of memory processing. Multimodal imaging during sleep may also provide important information regarding brain behavior during different states of arousal with different oscillatory properties[163, 164]. Findings from these future studies will aid in the interpretation of results from work utilizing a single neuroimaging technique or research focused on a specific cortical region.

Interpretation of CE results may have also been limited by the number of TMS-evoked measures elicited for each measurement at each assessment. The number of stimulation pulses delivered at each assessment were less than reported in other TMS studies of cortical excitability and may have affected the reliability of the response[114, 165, 166]. However, this is unlikely as the stability of measurement for SP MEP and CSP was discussed above and a related study observed significant changes in SP MEP and PP ratios with only seven trials collected for each measure[153]. Additionally, priming effects of one stimulation paradigm on another may have modulated the evoked responses. To control for this effect, we collected SP MEP data before and after PP MEP data collection. Also, we maintained the same order of CE tests within an assessment across each assessment, therefore, if one paradigm significantly influenced another, this effect would have been accounted for by maintaining the temporal relationships across assessments. Future work could further randomize stimulation paradigms such as interspersing SP MEP trials within PP MEP trials or combining CSP trials with SP/PP data collection. This would randomize active and passive conditions of the target muscle to further control for any potential order effects influencing TMS-evoked measures of cortical excitability.

Although no differences were found for the majority of CE measurements, results do indicate stability and repeatability of these measures over time. A common limitation of TMS-evoked measurements of CE is the variability of the outcome measurements, primarily SP MEP[106]. Here, SP MEPs were collected using ~1mVT in order to minimize potential floor and ceiling effects for PP MEP ratio calculation[111]. Mean SP MEP values for each group at each assessment were consistently near 1mV (Figure 11). This suggests that utilization of 1mVT as a test stimulation intensity to elicit SP MEPs is a stable, repeatable technique to elicit responses with minimal variability. This TMS-evoked EMG response stability was also observed for CSP measurement where significant changes in duration were not observed at any assessment for either group. In summary, limited changes in CE were observed but TMS-evoked measures of CE demonstrate stability across assessments with the stimulation parameters used. Therefore, future investigations can utilize these TMS parameters and combine with other neuroimaging techniques to comprehensively evaluate the neural mechanisms underlying motor skill learning and the role sleep plays in these neural processes

3. Objective sleep quality following training was predictive of the level of skill performance in the next follow-up skill assessment and a differential effect of task complexity was observed between training groups.

To date, this is the first study to examine the role of sleep prior to, and following, motor skill learning using actigraphy. Actigraphy is a low-cost, easy to administer method of sleep quality assessment. It also affords the benefit of sleep assessment in normal environments rather than a sleep research lab. While it is unable to measure specific sleep stages, it can quantify salient parameter of sleep such as, time to sleep, time asleep, time awake and number of times awake. For these characteristics of sleep, actigraphy has shown excellent agreement with PSG[96, 99]. Here, actigraphic assessment of sleep did not demonstrate a difference in pre-training sleep quality on the night before the initial visit, nor were there differences observed between the training groups for the second night once the skill had been acquired. These findings are in line with previous work using high-density EEG to measure global and local oscillatory changes in electrical activity of the brain following skill training[67, 70, 79].

Huber and colleagues[79] demonstrated that overall sleep architecture does not change following motor skill training but using a 256-electrode high-density EEG, they were able to demonstrate changes in local slow wave sleep activity during stage 3 and 4 sleep in the primary sensorimotor cortices contralateral to the trained hand. Actigraphy does not have the degree of spatial or temporal resolution of high-density EEG but data are in agreement with this technique for post-training changes in general sleep architecture. An interesting finding herein is the significant relationship observed between level of sleep quality and subsequent tracking performance.

Prior to training, actigraphic measures of sleep quality were not associated with initial finger-tracking performance in either training group, but at 12hr follow-up, performance was linked with sleep quality of the previous night in both groups. When subjects trained at night, the quality of sleep was predictive of the variance in performance the following morning, specifically for the S-R incompatible tracking condition. Although, data suggests that reduced sleep quality was associated with better skill performance in this group for incompatible tracking. Conversely, when training occurred in the morning and subjects returned after a twelve-hour interval of waking activity, sleep quality was predictive of S-R compatible tracking skill performance. In this case, greater sleep quality was associated with better performance. It is difficult to compare these results directly based on the timing differences between the night of sleep measured and the assessment point for skill performance, but these results demonstrate an observable relationship between sleep and skill development.

There is the potential that reduced sleep quality in the night group obscured other processes occurring during a sleep episode. As discussed previously, actigraphy lacks spatial specificity of cortical processes occurring during sleep[96, 99]. It also has poor resolution to measure changes in specific sleep stages. Therefore, broad changes in sleep architecture indicating diminished sleep quality may have occurred before or after information processing in specific cortical regions. This is speculative and was not a primary aim of this paper. Further work is warranted to replicate these findings and measure actigraphic sleep quality compared with gold standard PSG to comprehensively evaluate the relationship between sleep quality and finger-tracking skill performance.

In the day training group, the positive relationship between sleep quality the night prior to training and S-R compatible tracking performance at 12hr follow-up assessment during the following evening may have been related to level of arousal and alertness since there was no observable relationship between this sleep epoch and the significant improvement in performance from post-training to follow-up. Yet, subjective level of arousal was not different at this time point. As discussed above, the training paradigm attempted to account for time of day effects in skill performance over time and the results suggest that these confounds were adequately controlled. Despite the lack of a relationship between preceding night sleep quality and change in performance, these data do demonstrate a beneficial link between sleep quality measured by actigraphy and subsequent finger tracking performance after training.

Although sleep quality was not related to immediate offline skill improvements, it was predictive of the change in performance in tracking accuracy for the S-R compatible condition one day after training in the day training group. This finding should be interpreted cautiously since performance at 24hr follow-up was not significantly different than performance during the 12hr follow-up assessment the preceding evening. Again, these data may indicate solely performance improvements due to improved alertness and arousal levels secondary to better sleep quality the previous night. This is unlikely as tracking performance at this assessment was not significantly related to sleep quality; rather, the individual change in skill over the preceding 24hrs was associated with sleep. While interpretation is guarded, these preliminary findings indicate that sleep quality the night following training may be an important factor to consider in the evaluation of subsequent skill performance, at least for the next day. These results also invite follow-up investigation using other motor skills such as the SRTT or dynamic adaptation tasks to evaluate the relationship between sleep quality with skill performance and offline skill development.

4. No significant differences in skill development were found between skilled tracking training and simple, repeated movement.

The lack of a robust training effect for the training protocol compared with an equivalent period of repeated, unskilled movement may have been a result of multiple factors. First, the lack of effect between skilled and unskilled training could be indicative of substantial skill acquisition occurring within the skill assessments alone. This could be contributed to features of the test waveform. The triangle waveform contains a rhythmic component and was presented at an average fixed frequency and does not require abrupt directional changes compared with other waveforms. Also, the same waveform was presented repeatedly during each assessment, therefore, all subjects received ten exposures to the test waveform which may have been sufficient to trigger significant skill acquisition and memory consolidation[129]. If this were the case, the assumption would be that for the training groups, the skill was rapidly acquired during the assessment repetitions and the training practice may have made minimal contributions to skill development over the subsequent twenty-four hours. Also, long-term skill retention was not assessed in this design and may have been a useful indicator of skill learning as a result of training.

Regarding the rate of improvement, visual inspection of the performance curves between the groups suggests that training modifies the slope of the curve, creating a faster learning process. The results appear to indicate that asymptotic performance occurred earlier after training than after simply moving (Figure 23). This is the case only for the S-R compatible task, where there is a steep increase in skill performance from pre- to post-training with a small, but significant, gain in skill at follow-up. Whereas, in the movement group, the slope was relatively constant indicating consistent increases in performance at each assessment. It is important to note that these relationships do not appear to be the result of a within-assessment training effect for the training groups since the only significant difference in trial performance for a given assessment was at pre-training. Interestingly, these results were not observed for the incompatible condition. It was hypothesized that skilled training would have preferentially benefitted this condition since it requires greater perceptual processing to resolve the conflicting visual and proprioceptive input. One rationale may have been the training paradigm design. The majority of conditions during training were S-R compatible (80%); therefore, there was substantially greater exposure to the compatible condition across a variety of test conditions than the incompatible condition. If this were the case, potential learning effects due to the training period may have been limited in scope.

The experimental design did not specifically test skill transfer or generalizability to a related motor skill. The primary features of skill learning are repeatability and transferability[13, 14]. Here, repeatability of skilled performance was demonstrated up to one day following training. It could be argued that task transfer was partially probed by inclusion of the S-R incompatible condition, which was practiced only 20% of the training period. This was not a focus of the research design but in comparing the performance curves between the tracking and movement groups, it raises interesting questions about the degree of benefit afforded by the training period.

The training period here was brief and may not have been sufficient to promote substantive neural changes beyond those produced from the assessments alone. In a number of animal models, a high number of repetitions have been shown to be necessary to promote neural plasticity and cortical reorganization[23, 24, 167] associated with observed skill learning. In humans, hundreds of trials may be necessary to learn a skill[168]. Recently, in neurologically impaired humans, it has been theorized that approximately 400 repetitions may be necessary for significant cortical reorganization[169]. During each assessment, subjects performed six complete skilled flexion/extension movements each trial. Therefore, during each assessment alone, sixty movements were performed, whereas, during the training period, in excess of 800 skilled flexion/extension movements were performed. In the movement group, the same number of movements were performed but visuospatial feedback and feedforward information was not provided. Based on recommended repetitions for functional activities, the number of repetitions performed in the assessment phases may have been sufficient for the skill to be learned[168]. Whereas, the additional skilled tracking repetitions during training may have been insufficient to produce significant added improvement once asymptotic performance had been reached. Future research may administer repeated training sessions to promote further gains in performance. Alternatively, studies may also eliminate the training period altogether as these results indicate that significantly fewer repetitions may be sufficient to induce changes in skill performance that last at least one day.

VI. Conclusions

These results demonstrate that young, healthy individuals rapidly acquire proficiency for a continuous, goal-directed visuospatial skill that is not only retained over a period of time including sleep but also an interval consisting of normal, waking activity. These findings were in contrast to the initial hypotheses of the study but recent sleep and motor learning literature support the observed findings. Changes in skill performance were associated with neural activity and sleep quality, but only after training had occurred. Also, results did not demonstrate a substantial benefit of a twenty-minute skill training session compared to simple movement alone.

These data are in line with recent investigations demonstrating a limited role for sleep in post-training information processing in young, healthy individuals. Interestingly, both implicit and explicit versions of a continuous tracking skill, similar to the one employed in this study, were enhanced by sleep following training for individuals with chronic stroke[47, 71]. Also, sleep-dependent gains in sequential motor skill learning have been observed for subjects with prefrontal lobe lesions[170]. These results are encouraging but neither investigated the neural mechanisms underlying these observations, nor was sleep objectively quantified.

The conclusions drawn from this work, combined with related studies in patient populations, provide a foundation to evaluate the relationship between sleep, changes in neural activity, and the time course of continuous visuospatial motor skill learning in individuals following neurologic insult. The improved understanding of these processes and relationships from this work in healthy individuals now provides normative data to compare to future results in neurologic patient populations. Continuing this line of inquiry will ultimately provide a comprehensive evaluation of the therapeutic potential of sleep that will inform future rehabilitation paradigms in an effort to maximize skill (re)learning and restoration of function following neurologic injury.

VII. References

1. Maquet, P. The role of sleep in learning and memory. *Science* **294**, 1048-1052 (2001).
2. Peigneux, P., Laureys, S., Delbeuck, X. & Maquet, P. Sleeping brain, learning brain. The role of sleep for memory systems. *Neuroreport* **12**, A111-124 (2001).
3. Cirelli, C. A molecular window on sleep: changes in gene expression between sleep and wakefulness. *Neuroscientist* **11**, 63-74 (2005).
4. Tononi, G. & Cirelli, C. Sleep function and synaptic homeostasis. *Sleep Medicine Reviews* **10**, 49-62 (2006).
5. Walker, M.P. & Stickgold, R. Sleep, memory, and plasticity. *Annual Review of Psychology* **57**, 139-166 (2006).
6. Tononi, G. & Cirelli, C. Some considerations on sleep and neural plasticity. *Archives Italiennes de Biologie* **139**, 221-241 (2001).
7. Walker, M.P., Brakefield, T., Morgan, A., Hobson, J.A. & Stickgold, R. Practice with sleep makes perfect: sleep-dependent motor skill learning.[see comment]. *Neuron* **35**, 205-211 (2002).
8. Fogel, S.M., Nader, R., Cote, K.A. & Smith, C.T. Sleep spindles and learning potential. *Behavioral Neuroscience* **121**, 1-10 (2007).
9. Walker, M.P., *et al.* Sleep and the time course of motor skill learning. *Learning & Memory* **10**, 275-284 (2003).
10. Stickgold, R., Whidbee, D., Schirmer, B., Patel, V. & Hobson, J.A. Visual discrimination task improvement: A multi-step process occurring during sleep. *Journal of Cognitive Neuroscience* **12**, 246-254 (2000).
11. Kuriyama, K., Stickgold, R. & Walker, M.P. Sleep-dependent learning and motor-skill complexity. *Learning & Memory* **11**, 705-713 (2004).
12. Fischer, S., Hallschmid, M., Elsner, A.L. & Born, J. Sleep forms memory for finger skills. *Proceedings of the National Academy of Sciences of the United States of America* **99**, 11987-11991 (2002).
13. Shumway-Cook, A.W., Marjorie J. *Motor Control - Translating Research into Clinical Practice* (Lippincott Williams & Wilkins, Baltimore, 2007).
14. Schmidt RA, L.T. *Motor Control and Learning: A Behavioral Emphasis* (Human Kinetics, Champaign, IL, 2005).
15. Winstein, C. Designing practice for motor learning: clinical implications: contemporary menagement of motor control problems. in *Proceedings of the II Step Conference* (Alexandria, VA, 1991).
16. Hird, J., Landers, D., Thomas, J. & Horan, J. Physical practice is superior to mental practice in enhancing cognitive and motor task performance. *Journal of Sport and Exercise Psychology* **13**, 281-293. (1991).
17. Eysnek HJ, F.C. *Reminiscence, motivation, and personality: A case study in experimental psychology* (Plenum Press, New York & London, 1977).
18. Robertson, E.M., Pascual-Leone, A. & Miall, R.C. Current concepts in procedural consolidation. *Nature Reviews Neuroscience* **5**, 576-582 (2004).
19. Rioult-Pedotti, M.S., Friedman, D. & Donoghue, J.P. Learning-induced LTP in neocortex. *Science* **290**, 533-536 (2000).

20. Stefan, K., *et al.* Temporary occlusion of associative motor cortical plasticity by prior dynamic motor training. *Cerebral Cortex* **16**, 376-385 (2006).
21. Ziemann, U., *et al.* Learning modifies subsequent induction of long-term potentiation-like and long-term depression-like plasticity in human motor cortex.[erratum appears in J Neurosci. 2004 Nov 17;24(46):1 p following 10552 Note: Iliac, Tihomir V [corrected to Ilic, Tihomir V]]. *Journal of Neuroscience* **24**, 1666-1672 (2004).
22. Elbert, T., Pantev, C., Wienbruch, C., Rockstroh, B. & Taub, E. Increased cortical representation of the fingers of the left hand in string players. *Science* **270**, 305-307 (1995).
23. Nudo, R., Milliken, G., Jenkins, W. & Merzenich, M. Use-dependent alterations of movement representations in primary motor cortex of adult squirrel monkeys. *J Neurosci* **16(2)**, 785-807 (1996).
24. Plautz, E.J., Milliken, G.W. & Nudo, R.J. Effects of repetitive motor training on movement representations in adult squirrel monkeys: role of use versus learning. *Neurobiology of Learning and Memory* **74**, 27-55 (2000).
25. Carey, J.R., *et al.* Primary Motor Area Activation during Precision-Demanding versus Simple Finger Movement. *Neurorehabilitation & Neural Repair* **20**, 361-370 (2006).
26. Shadmehr, R. & Krakauer, J.W. A computational neuroanatomy for motor control. *Experimental Brain Research* **185**, 359-381 (2008).
27. Soechting, J.F., Flanders, M., Soechting, J.F. & Flanders, M. Sensorimotor control of contact force. *Current Opinion in Neurobiology* **18**, 565-572 (2008).
28. Kording, K.P., *et al.* Bayesian integration in force estimation. *Journal of Neurophysiology* **92**, 3161-3165 (2004).
29. Kording, K.P., *et al.* A neuroeconomics approach to inferring utility functions in sensorimotor control. *Plos Biology* **2**, e330 (2004).
30. Kandel, E., Schwartz, J. & Jessell, T. *Principles of neural science* (McGraw-Hill, New York, 2000).
31. Cahill, L., *et al.* Amygdala activity at encoding correlated with long-term, free recall of emotional information. *Proceedings of the National Academy of Sciences of the United States of America* **93**, 8016-8021 (1996).
32. Schmidt, R.A., Young, D.E., Swinnen, S. & Shapiro, D.C. Summary knowledge of results for skill acquisition: support for the guidance hypothesis. *Journal of Experimental Psychology: Learning, Memory, & Cognition* **15**, 352-359 (1989).
33. Winstein CJ, S.R. Reduced frequency of knowledge of results enhances motor skill learning. *Journal of Experimental Psychology: Learning, Memory, & Cognition* **16**, 14 (1990).
34. Boyd, L.A. The interaction between explicit knowledge and implicit motor-sequence learning following focal brain damage. **286** (2001).
35. Boyd, L.A. & Winstein, C.J. Impact of explicit information on implicit motor-sequence learning following middle cerebral artery stroke. *Physical Therapy* **83**, 976-989 (2003).
36. Boyd, L.A. & Winstein, C.J. Providing explicit information disrupts implicit motor learning after basal ganglia stroke. *Learning & Memory* **11**, 388-396 (2004).

37. Boyd, L.A. & Winstein, C.J. Explicit information interferes with implicit motor learning of both continuous and discrete movement tasks after stroke. *Journal of Neurologic Physical Therapy* **30**, 46-59 (2006).
38. Walker, M.P. A refined model of sleep and the time course of memory formation. *Behavioral & Brain Sciences* **28**, 51-64; discussion 64-104 (2005).
39. Robertson, E.M., Pascual-Leone, A. & Press, D.Z. Awareness modifies the skill-learning benefits of sleep. *Current Biology* **14**, 208-212 (2004).
40. Song, S., et al. Sleep does not benefit probabilistic motor sequence learning. *Journal of Neuroscience* **27**, 12475-12483 (2007).
41. Krakauer, J.W. & Shadmehr, R. Consolidation of motor memory. *Trends in Neurosciences* **29**, 58-64 (2006).
42. Walker, M.P., Stickgold, R., Alsop, D., Gaab, N. & Schlaug, G. Sleep-dependent motor memory plasticity in the human brain. *Neuroscience* **133**, 911-917 (2005).
43. Walker, M.P., Brakefield, T., Hobson, J.A. & Stickgold, R. Dissociable stages of human memory consolidation and reconsolidation.[see comment]. *Nature* **425**, 616-620 (2003).
44. Doyon, J., et al. Contribution of night and day sleep vs. simple passage of time to the consolidation of motor sequence and visuomotor adaptation learning. *Experimental Brain Research* **195**, 15-26 (2009).
45. Baraduc, P., Lang, N., Rothwell, J.C. & Wolpert, D.M. Consolidation of dynamic motor learning is not disrupted by rTMS of primary motor cortex. *Current Biology* **14**, 252-256 (2004).
46. Hadipour-Niktarash, A., et al. Impairment of retention but not acquisition of a visuomotor skill through time-dependent disruption of primary motor cortex. *Journal of Neuroscience* **27**, 13413-13419 (2007).
47. Siengsukon, C., Boyd, L.A., Siengsukon, C. & Boyd, L.A. Sleep enhances off-line spatial and temporal motor learning after stroke. *Neurorehabilitation & Neural Repair* **23**, 327-335 (2009).
48. Boyd, L.A., et al. Motor sequence chunking is impaired by basal ganglia stroke. *Neurobiology of Learning & Memory* **92**, 35-44 (2009).
49. Carey, J.R., et al. Tracking vs. movement telerehabilitation training to change hand function and brain reorganization in stroke. *Neurorehabilitation & Neural Repair* (in press).
50. Carey, J., Baxter, T. & Di Fabio, R. Tracking control in the nonparetic hand of subjects with stroke. *Arch Phys Med Rehabil* **79**, 435-441 (1998).
51. Carey, J.R., et al. fMRI analysis of ankle movement tracking training in subject with stroke. *Exp Brain Res* **54**, 281-290 (2004).
52. Carey, J.R., et al. Comparison of finger tracking versus simple movement training via telerehabilitation to alter hand function and cortical reorganization after stroke. *Neurorehabilitation & Neural Repair* **21**, 216-232 (2007).
53. Borich, M. Goal-directed visuomotor skill learning: off-line enhancement and the importance of the primary motor cortex. *Restorative Neurology & Neuroscience* (in press).

54. Squire, L.R. & Zola, S.M. Structure and function of declarative and nondeclarative memory systems. *Proceedings of the National Academy of Sciences of the United States of America* **93**, 13515-13522 (1996).
55. Squire, L.R. Memory and the hippocampus: a synthesis from findings with rats, monkeys, and humans. *Psychological Review* **99**, 195-231 (1992).
56. McGaugh, J.L. Memory--a century of consolidation. *Science* **287**, 248-251 (2000).
57. Cohen, D.A., Pascual-Leone, A., Press, D.Z. & Robertson, E.M. Off-line learning of motor skill memory: a double dissociation of goal and movement. *Proceedings of the National Academy of Sciences of the United States of America* **102**, 18237-18241 (2005).
58. Cohen, D.A. & Robertson, E.M. Motor sequence consolidation: constrained by critical time windows or competing components. *Experimental Brain Research* **177**, 440-446 (2007).
59. Brashers-Krug, T., Shadmehr, R. & Bizzi, E. Consolidation in human motor memory. *Nature* **382**, 252-255 (1996).
60. Robertson, E.M., Press, D.Z. & Pascual-Leone, A. Off-line learning and the primary motor cortex.[see comment]. *Journal of Neuroscience* **25**, 6372-6378 (2005).
61. Sanes, J. & Donoghue, J. Plasticity and primary motor cortex [Review]. *Annual Review Neuroscience* **23**, 393-415 (2000).
62. Hebb, D.O. *The Organization of Behavior* (Wiley & Sons, New York, 1949).
63. Benington, J.H. & Frank, M.G. Cellular and molecular connections between sleep and synaptic plasticity. *Progress in Neurobiology* **69**, 71-101 (2003).
64. Jay, T.M. & Jay, T.M. Dopamine: a potential substrate for synaptic plasticity and memory mechanisms. *Progress in Neurobiology* **69**, 375-390 (2003).
65. Ungerleider, L.G., Doyon, J. & Karni, A. Imaging brain plasticity during motor skill learning. *Neurobiology of Learning & Memory* **78**, 553-564 (2002).
66. Mushiake, H., Inase, M. & Tanji, J. Neuronal activity in the primate premotor, supplementary, and precentral motor cortex during visually guided and internally determined sequential movements. *Journal of Neurophysiology* **66**, 705-718 (1991).
67. Huber, R., et al. Arm immobilization causes cortical plastic changes and locally decreases sleep slow wave activity. *Nature Neuroscience* **9**, 1169-1176 (2006).
68. Huber, R., et al. Measures of cortical plasticity after transcranial paired associative stimulation predict changes in electroencephalogram slow-wave activity during subsequent sleep. *Journal of Neuroscience* **28**, 7911-7918 (2008).
69. Vyazovskiy, V.V., Cirelli, C., Pfister-Genskow, M., Faraguna, U. & Tononi, G. Molecular and electrophysiological evidence for net synaptic potentiation in wake and depression in sleep.[see comment]. *Nature Neuroscience* **11**, 200-208 (2008).
70. Huber, R., et al. TMS-induced cortical potentiation during wakefulness locally increases slow wave activity during sleep. *PLoS ONE [Electronic Resource]* **2**, e276 (2007).
71. Siengsukon, C.F. & Boyd, L.A. Sleep enhances implicit motor skill learning in individuals poststroke. *Topics in Stroke Rehabilitation* **15**, 1-12 (2008).

72. Hikosaka, O., Miyasita, K., Miyachi, S., Sakai, K. & Lu, X. Differential roles of the frontal cortex, basal ganglia and cerebellum in visuomotor sequence learning. *Neurobiol Learn Mem* **70**, 137-149 (1998).
73. Hikosaka, O., Nakamura, K., Sakai, K. & Nakahara, H. Central mechanisms of motor skill learning. *Current Opinion in Neurobiology* **12**, 217-222 (2002).
74. Goedert, K.M., Willingham, D.B., Goedert, K.M. & Willingham, D.B. Patterns of interference in sequence learning and prism adaptation inconsistent with the consolidation hypothesis. *Learning & Memory* **9**, 279-292 (2002).
75. Tucker, M.A., *et al.* A daytime nap containing solely non-REM sleep enhances declarative but not procedural memory. *Neurobiology of Learning & Memory* **86**, 241-247 (2006).
76. Karni, A., Tanne, D., Rubenstein, B.S., Askenasy, J.J. & Sagi, D. Dependence on REM sleep of overnight improvement of a perceptual skill.[see comment]. *Science* **265**, 679-682 (1994).
77. Stickgold, R., James, L. & Hobson, J.A. Visual discrimination learning requires sleep after training.[see comment]. *Nature Neuroscience* **3**, 1237-1238 (2000).
78. Bergmann, T.O., *et al.* A local signature of LTP- and LTD-like plasticity in human NREM sleep. *European Journal of Neuroscience* **27**, 2241-2249 (2008).
79. Huber, R., Ghilardi, M.F., Massimini, M. & Tononi, G. Local sleep and learning.[see comment]. *Nature* **430**, 78-81 (2004).
80. Marshall, L., *et al.* Boosting slow oscillations during sleep potentiates memory.[see comment]. *Nature* **444**, 610-613 (2006).
81. Borbely, A.A. From slow waves to sleep homeostasis: new perspectives. *Archives Italiennes de Biologie* **139**, 53-61 (2001).
82. Bal, T. & McCormick, D.A. Synchronized oscillations in the inferior olive are controlled by the hyperpolarization-activated cation current I(h). *Journal of Neurophysiology* **77**, 3145-3156 (1997).
83. Benington, J.H., Frank, M.G., Benington, J.H. & Frank, M.G. Cellular and molecular connections between sleep and synaptic plasticity. *Progress in Neurobiology* **69**, 71-101 (2003).
84. Steriade, M., Timofeev, I., Steriade, M. & Timofeev, I. Neuronal plasticity in thalamocortical networks during sleep and waking oscillations. *Neuron* **37**, 563-576 (2003).
85. Kemp, N. & Bashir, Z.I. Long-term depression: a cascade of induction and expression mechanisms. *Progress in Neurobiology* **65**, 339-365 (2001).
86. Cirelli, C. & Tononi, G. Gene expression in the brain across the sleep-waking cycle. *Brain Research* **885**, 303-321 (2000).
87. Tononi, G. & Cirelli, C. Sleep and synaptic homeostasis: a hypothesis. *Brain Research Bulletin* **62**, 143-150 (2003).
88. Maquet, P., *et al.* Experience-dependent changes in cerebral activation during human REM sleep. *Nature Neuroscience* **3**, 831-836 (2000).
89. Gais, S., *et al.* Visual-procedural memory consolidation during sleep blocked by glutamatergic receptor antagonists. *Journal of Neuroscience* **28**, 5513-5518 (2008).

90. Buysse, D.J., Reynolds, C.F., 3rd, Monk, T.H., Berman, S.R. & Kupfer, D.J. The Pittsburgh Sleep Quality Index: a new instrument for psychiatric practice and research. *Psychiatry Research* **28**, 193-213 (1989).

91. Johns, M.W. A new method for measuring daytime sleepiness: the Epworth sleepiness scale. *Sleep* **14**, 540-545 (1991).

92. Hoddes, E., Zarcone, V., Smythe, H., Phillips, R. & Dement, W.C. Quantification of sleepiness: a new approach. *Psychophysiology* **10**, 431-436 (1973).

93. Buysse, D.J., *et al.* Relationships between the Pittsburgh Sleep Quality Index (PSQI), Epworth Sleepiness Scale (ESS), and clinical/polysomnographic measures in a community sample. *Journal of Clinical Sleep Medicine* **4**, 563-571 (2008).

94. Kushida, C.A., *et al.* Practice parameters for the indications for polysomnography and related procedures: an update for 2005. *Sleep* **28**, 499-521 (2005).

95. Zollman, F.S., *et al.* Actigraphy for assessment of sleep in traumatic brain injury: case series, review of the literature and proposed criteria for use. *Brain Injury* **24**, 748-754 (2010).

96. Acebo, C., LeBourgeois, M.K., Acebo, C. & LeBourgeois, M.K. Actigraphy. *Respiratory Care Clinics of North America* **12**, 23-30 (2006).

97. Berger, A.M., *et al.* Methodological challenges when using actigraphy in research. *Journal of Pain & Symptom Management* **36**, 191-199 (2008).

98. Morgenthaler, T., *et al.* Practice parameters for the use of actigraphy in the assessment of sleep and sleep disorders: an update for 2007. *Sleep* **30**, 519-529 (2007).

99. Weiss, A.R., *et al.* Validity of activity-based devices to estimate sleep. *Journal of Clinical Sleep Medicine* **6**, 336-342 (2010).

100. Sadeh, A., Hauri, P.J., Kripke, D.F. & Lavie, P. The role of actigraphy in the evaluation of sleep disorders. *Sleep* **18**, 288-302 (1995).

101. Beecroft, J.M., *et al.* Sleep monitoring in the intensive care unit: comparison of nurse assessment, actigraphy and polysomnography. *Intensive Care Medicine* **34**, 2076-2083 (2008).

102. Carney, C.E., *et al.* Wrist actigraph versus self-report in normal sleepers: sleep schedule adherence and self-report validity. *Behavioral Sleep Medicine* **2**, 134-143; discussion 144-137 (2004).

103. Alessi, C.A., Yoon, E.J., Schnelle, J.F., Al-Samarrai, N.R. & Cruise, P.A. A randomized trial of a combined physical activity and environmental intervention in nursing home residents: do sleep and agitation improve? *Journal of the American Geriatrics Society* **47**, 784-791 (1999).

104. Van Someren, E.J., Lijzenga, C., Mirmiran, M. & Swaab, D.F. Long-term fitness training improves the circadian rest-activity rhythm in healthy elderly males. *Journal of Biological Rhythms* **12**, 146-156 (1997).

105. Hallett, M. Dystonia: abnormal movements result from loss of inhibition. *Advances in Neurology* **94**, 1-9 (2004).

106. Wassermann, E.M. *The Oxford Handbook of Transcranial Stimulation* (Oxford University Press, 2008).

107. Barker, A.T. The history and basic principles of magnetic nerve stimulation. *Electroencephalography & Clinical Neurophysiology - Supplement* **51**, 3-21 (1999).

108. Nollet, H., Van Ham, L., Deprez, P. & Vanderstraeten, G. Transcranial magnetic stimulation: review of the technique, basic principles and applications. *Veterinary Journal* **166**, 28-42 (2003).
109. Ruohonen, J. & Ilmoniemi, R.J. Modeling of the stimulating field generation in TMS. *Electroencephalography & Clinical Neurophysiology - Supplement* **51**, 30-40 (1999).
110. Rossini, P.M., et al. Applications of magnetic cortical stimulation. The International Federation of Clinical Neurophysiology. *Electroencephalography & Clinical Neurophysiology - Supplement* **52**, 171-185 (1999).
111. Sanger, T.D., Garg, R.R. & Chen, R. Interactions between two different inhibitory systems in the human motor cortex. *Journal of Physiology* **530**, 307-317 (2001).
112. Sparing, R., Buelte, D., Meister, I.G., Paus, T. & Fink, G.R. Transcranial magnetic stimulation and the challenge of coil placement: a comparison of conventional and stereotaxic neuronavigational strategies. *Human Brain Mapping* **29**, 82-96 (2008).
113. Sparing, R., et al. Transcranial magnetic stimulation and the challenge of coil placement: a comparison of conventional and stereotaxic neuronavigational strategies. *Human Brain Mapping* **29**, 82-96 (2008).
114. Gangitano, M., et al. Modulation of input-output curves by low and high frequency repetitive transcranial magnetic stimulation of the motor cortex. *Clinical Neurophysiology* **113**, 1249-1257 (2002).
115. Ziemann, U., Lonnecker, S., Steinhoff, B.J. & Paulus, W. The effect of lorazepam on the motor cortical excitability in man. *Experimental Brain Research* **109**, 127-135 (1996).
116. Kujirai, T., et al. Corticocortical inhibition in human motor cortex. *Journal of Physiology* **471**, 501-519 (1993).
117. Ziemann, U., Rothwell, J.C. & Ridding, M.C. Interaction between intracortical inhibition and facilitation in human motor cortex. *Journal of Physiology* **496**, 873-881 (1996).
118. Siebner, H.R. & Rothwell, J. Transcranial magnetic stimulation: new insights into representational cortical plasticity. *Exp Brain Res* **148**, 1-16 (2003).
119. Chen, R., et al. Depression of motor cortex excitability by low-frequency transcranial magnetic stimulation. *Neurology* **48**, 1398-1403 (1997).
120. Pascual-Leone, A., Valls-Sole, J., Wassermann, E.M. & Hallett, M. Responses to rapid-rate transcranial magnetic stimulation of the human motor cortex. *Brain* **117**, 847-858 (1994).
121. Ljubisavljevic, M., Kacar, A., Milanovic, S., Svetel, M. & Kostic, V.S. Changes in cortical inhibition during task-specific contractions in primary writing tremor patients. *Movement Disorders* **21**, 855-859 (2006).
122. Muellbacher, W., Ziemann, U., Boroojerdi, B., Cohen, L. & Hallett, M. Role of the human motor cortex in rapid motor learning. *Experimental Brain Research* **136**, 431-438 (2001).
123. Muellbacher, W., et al. Early consolidation in human primary motor cortex. *Nature* **415**, 640-644 (2002).

124. Smith, C., Smith, D., Smith, C. & Smith, D. Ingestion of ethanol just prior to sleep onset impairs memory for procedural but not declarative tasks. *Sleep* **26**, 185-191 (2003).
125. Oldfield, R. The assessment and analysis of handedness: the Edinburgh inventory. *Neuropsychologia* **9(1)**, 97-113 (1971).
126. Rosler, K.M., et al. Effect of discharge desynchronization on the size of motor evoked potentials: an analysis. *Clinical Neurophysiology* **113**, 1680-1687 (2002).
127. Wassermann, E.M. & Lisanby, S.H. Therapeutic application of repetitive transcranial magnetic stimulation: a review. *Clinical Neurophysiology* **112**, 1367-1377 (2001).
128. Carey, J.R., et al. Analysis of fMRI and Finger Tracking Training in Subjects with Chronic Stroke. *Brain* **125**, 773-788 (2002).
129. Carey, J.R., Fregni, F. & Pascual-Leone, A. rTMS combined with motor learning training in healthy subjects. *Restorative Neurology & Neuroscience* **24**, 191-199 (2006).
130. Carey, J., Bogard, C., Youdas, J. & Suman, V. Stimulus-response compatibility effects in a manual tracking task. *Percept Mot Skills* **81**, 1155-1170 (1995).
131. Moran, D.W. & Schwartz, A.B. Motor cortical representation of speed and direction during reaching. *Journal of Neurophysiology* **82**, 2676-2692 (1999).
132. Carey, J. Manual stretch: Effect on finger movement control and force control in subjects with stroke with spastic extrinsic finger flexor muscles. *Arch Phys Med Rehabil* **71**, 888-894 (1990).
133. Robertson, E.M., Cohen, D.A., Robertson, E.M. & Cohen, D.A. Understanding consolidation through the architecture of memories. *Neuroscientist* **12**, 261-271 (2006).
134. Maeda, F., et al. Inter- and intra-individual variability of paired-pulse curves with transcranial magnetic stimulation (TMS). *Clinical Neurophysiology* **113**, 376-382 (2002).
135. Kimberley, T.J., et al. Establishing the definition and inter-rater reliability of cortical silent period calculation in subjects with focal hand dystonia and healthy controls. *Neuroscience Letters* **464**, 84-87 (2009).
136. Sadeh, A., Sharkey, K.M. & Carskadon, M.A. Activity-based sleep-wake identification: an empirical test of methodological issues. *Sleep* **17**, 201-207 (1994).
137. Short, M., et al. Does subjective sleepiness predict objective sleep propensity? *Sleep* **33**, 123-129.
138. Newman, J. & Broughton, R. Pupillometric assessment of excessive daytime sleepiness in narcolepsy-cataplexy. *Sleep* **14**, 121-129 (1991).
139. Johns, M.W. Sleepiness in different situations measured by the Epworth Sleepiness Scale. *Sleep* **17**, 703-710 (1994).
140. Portney, L. & Watkins, M. *Foundations of Clinical Research: Applications to Practice.* (Appleton & Lange, Norwalk, CN, 2000).
141. Field, A. *Discovering statistics using SPSS : (and sex, drugs and rock 'n' roll)* (Sage, London, 2009).
142. Howell, D.C. *Statistical Methods for Psychology* (Thomson Wadsworth, Belmont, California, 2007).

143. Bhatt, E., et al. Effect of finger tracking combined with electrical stimulation on brain reorganization and hand function in subjects with stroke. *Experimental Brain Research* **182**, 435-447 (2007).
144. Carey, J., Bogard, C., King, B. & Suman, V. Finger-movement tracking scores in healthy subjects. *Percept Mot Skills* **79**, 563-576 (1994).
145. Keisler, A., et al. Time of day accounts for overnight improvement in sequence learning. *Learning & Memory* **14**, 669-672 (2007).
146. Cai, D.J., Rickard, T.C., Cai, D.J. & Rickard, T.C. Reconsidering the role of sleep for motor memory. *Behavioral Neuroscience* **123**, 1153-1157 (2009).
147. G Matthews, R.D., SJ Westerman, RB Stammers. *Human Performance: Cognition, stress and individual differences.* (Taylor and Francis, Philadelphia, 2000).
148. Shadmehr, R. & Holcomb, H.H. Neural correlates of motor memory consolidation. *Science* **277**, 821-825 (1997).
149. Shadmehr, R. & Brashers-Krug, T. Functional stages in the formation of human long-term motor memory. *Journal of Neuroscience* **17**, 409-419 (1997).
150. Hotermans, C., et al. Repetitive transcranial magnetic stimulation over the primary motor cortex disrupts early boost but not delayed gains in performance in motor sequence learning. *European Journal of Neuroscience* **28**, 1216-1221 (2008).
151. Karni, A., et al. Functional MRI evidence for adult motor cortex plasticity during motor skill learning. *Nature* **377**, 155-158 (1995).
152. Classen, J., Liepert, J., Wise, S.P., Hallett, M. & Cohen, L.G. Rapid plasticity of human cortical movement representation induced by practice. *Journal of Neurophysiol* **79**, 1117-1123 (1998).
153. Gallasch, E., et al. Changes in motor cortex excitability following training of a novel goal-directed motor task. *European Journal of Applied Physiology* **105**, 47-54 (2009).
154. Ziemann, U., Muellbacher, W., Hallett, M. & Cohen, L.G. Modulation of practice-dependent plasticity in human motor cortex. *Brain* **124**, 1171-1181 (2001).
155. Floyer-Lea, A. & Matthews, P.M. Changing brain networks for visuomotor control with increased movement automaticity. *Journal of Neurophysiology* **92**, 2405-2412 (2004).
156. Koeneke, S., Lutz, K., Herwig, U., Ziemann, U. & Jancke, L. Extensive training of elementary finger tapping movements changes the pattern of motor cortex excitability. *Experimental Brain Research* **174**, 199-209 (2006).
157. Orban, P., et al. The multifaceted nature of the relationship between performance and brain activity in motor sequence learning. *Neuroimage* **49**, 694-702 (2010).
158. Hummel, F., et al. To act or not to act. Neural correlates of executive control of learned motor behavior. *Neuroimage* **23**, 1391-1401 (2004).
159. Siebner, H.R., et al. Consensus paper: combining transcranial stimulation with neuroimaging.[Erratum appears in Brain Stimul. 2009 Jul;2(3):182]. *Brain Stimulation* **2**, 58-80 (2009).
160. Gerloff, C., et al. Multimodal imaging of brain reorganization in motor areas of the contralesional hemisphere of well recovered patients after capsular stroke. *Brain* **129**, 791-808 (2006).

161. Fitzgerald, P.B. & Fitzgerald, P.B. TMS-EEG: a technique that has come of age? *Clinical Neurophysiology* **121**, 265-267 (2010).

162. Komssi, S., *et al.* Ipsi- and contralateral EEG reactions to transcranial magnetic stimulation. *Clinical Neurophysiology* **113**, 175-184 (2002).

163. Bergmann, T.O., *et al.* Acute changes in motor cortical excitability during slow oscillatory and constant anodal transcranial direct current stimulation. *Journal of Neurophysiology* **102**, 2303-2311 (2009).

164. Massimini, M., Tononi, G. & Huber, R. Slow waves, synaptic plasticity and information processing: insights from transcranial magnetic stimulation and high-density EEG experiments. *European Journal of Neuroscience* **29**, 1761-1770 (2009).

165. Schmidt, S., *et al.* An initial transient-state and reliable measures of corticospinal excitability in TMS studies. *Clinical Neurophysiology* **120**, 987-993 (2009).

166. Ortu, E., *et al.* Effects of volitional contraction on intracortical inhibition and facilitation in the human motor cortex. *Journal of Physiology* **586**, 5147-5159 (2008).

167. Kleim, J.A., Vij, K., Ballard, D.H. & Greenough, W.T. Learning-dependent synaptic modifications in the cerebellar cortex of the adult rat persist for at least four weeks. *Journal of Neuroscience.* **17**, 717-721 (1997).

168. Fine, M.S., Thoroughman, K.A., Fine, M.S. & Thoroughman, K.A. Motor adaptation to single force pulses: sensitive to direction but insensitive to within-movement pulse placement and magnitude. *Journal of Neurophysiology* **96**, 710-720 (2006).

169. Lang, C.E., *et al.* Observation of amounts of movement practice provided during stroke rehabilitation. *Archives of Physical Medicine & Rehabilitation* **90**, 1692-1698 (2009).

170. Gomez Beldarrain, M., *et al.* Sleep improves sequential motor learning and performance in patients with prefrontal lobe lesions. *Clinical Neurology & Neurosurgery* **110**, 245-252 (2008).

VIII. Appendices

Appendix A
Consent to Participate in Research Study:
Enhancement of learning: Does sleep benefit motor skill memory consolidation?

You are invited to participate in a research study investigating the effect of non-invasive brain stimulation using a device called a transcranial magnetic stimulator. You have been selected because you responded to a recruitment posting. This study is being conducted by Teresa J. Kimberley, PhD, PT, Sanjeev Arora, MD and Michael R Borich, DPT in the Program in Physical Therapy at the University Of Minnesota. We ask that you read this form and ask any questions you may have before agreeing to be in the study.

Study Purpose

The purpose of the study is to investigate the relationship between sleep and how motor skills are acquired by the brain. We are testing healthy adults in this study, and eventually would like to apply to persons who have had a stroke. We will test this by having subjects learn a skill before or after sleep and then reexamine skill performance after an interval with and without sleep. Also, brain activity will be studied using transcranial magnetic stimulation (TMS). By applying a magnetic field to the outside of the head, electrical currents are produced within the brain that can elicit a measurable response. Using this procedure, different areas of the brain can be studied to gain a greater understanding of the mechanisms associated with motor skill learning in healthy and patient populations.

Study Procedures

If you agree to participate, you will be seen for three visits. At the first visit, you will be asked about your health history, complete various brain and motor function tests. If you are a female of childbearing age, a pregnancy test will be administered by nursing staff at the General Clinical Research Center (GCRC). After this initial screening, you will be seated in a supportive chair and a swim cap will be applied to your head in order to make measurements and mark appropriate areas for brain stimulation. Also, small surface electrodes will be applied to your hand and connected to an EMG machine to record the electrical response of your finger muscle when stimulated. Your motor threshold will be measured by identifying the lowest intensity of stimulation required to produce a measurable response in your finger muscle. This is done by positioning a figure-of-8 coil over the area corresponding to the hand area of your brain. A very brief pulse of electric current will pass through the coil creating a localized magnetic field which can pass through the skull and activate the brain. A small tapping sensation may be felt on the scalp and a clicking noise will occur which will be minimized by ear plug usage. After each pulse, finger muscle activity will be assessed. Stimulus intensity and location will be systematically adjusted until the location is found which best produces a finger response using the lowest intensity of stimulation.

Next, you will be given a motor skill training program consisting of specific, repeated finger movements required to accurately track a pattern displayed on a computer screen. This will last for 20 minutes. Before and after training, measures of brain activity will be collected through stimulus application at a slightly higher intensity than used to identify your motor threshold. Finger muscle responses will be collected for each stimulus.

The second visit and third visit will consist of repeating the motor threshold identification procedure and the brain activity measurements conducted the previous day and will occur following an interval with or without sleep. You will be asked to keep a sleep journal and wear an activity monitor around your wrist while asleep for the nights prior to and following skill training. Total time for participation will be 2 hours for the first visit and 30 minutes each for the second and third visit.

Risks of Study Participation

There have been reports of a seizure from repetitive (r)TMS but no seizures have been reported with the TMS settings used in this study. Our procedure for managing a seizure includes:
- Presence in the area of a physician or nurse trained in seizure management
- Presence of, or ready access to, life support equipment (oxygen, suction, blood pressure monitor, cardio-pulmonary resuscitation (CPR) equipment)
- Access to anti-epileptic drugs

There is a social implication of seizure. A seizure can affect future employability, insurability, or eligibility to drive. To minimize this potential problem, we will provide to any subject who experiences a seizure a letter documenting that the seizure was experimentally produced.

The possibility exists for a temporary headache due to the TMS or the tight swim cap surrounding the head. There is also a risk for dental pain. If either of these pains occur, we will manage them by administering acetaminophen. The effects of TMS on thinking, memory and mood are not known. The effect of TMS on the unborn fetus is not known and participating women should not be pregnant. We may discontinue the treatment without your consent if we recognize any abnormal signals in muscle recordings or any abnormal behavioral responses.

Compensation for Injury

In the event that this research activity results in an injury, treatment will be available, including first aid, emergency treatment and follow-up care as needed. Care for such injuries will be billed in the ordinary manner, to you or your insurance company. If you think that you have suffered a research-related injury, please let us know right away.

Benefits of Study Participation

There is no direct benefit to you to participate in this study.

Study Costs/Compensation

There are no costs to you associated with this study. You will receive $10.00 for each visit, totaling $30.00 for completion of the study.

Confidentiality

The records of this study will be kept private. In any publications or presentations, we will not include any information that will make it possible to identify you as a subject. Your record for the study may, however, be reviewed by departments at the University with appropriate regulatory oversight. Each visit will be recorded on your Fairview medical record. To these extents, confidentiality is not absolute.

Protected Health Information (PHI)

Your PHI created or received for the purposes of this study is protected under the federal regulation known as HIPAA. Refer to the attached HIPAA authorization for details concerning the use of this information.

Voluntary Nature of the Study

Participation in this study is voluntary. Your decision whether or not to participate in this study will not affect your current or future relations with the University or the University of Minnesota Medical Center, Fairview. If you decide to participate, you are free to withdraw at any time without affecting those relationships.

Contacts and Questions

You may ask any questions you have now, or if you have questions later, you are encouraged to contact Teresa Kimberley at 612-626-4096 or Michael Borich at 612-626-0637.
If you have any questions or concerns regarding the study and would like to talk to someone other than the researcher(s), you are encouraged to contact the Fairview Research Helpline at telephone number 612-672-7692 or toll free at 866-508-6961. You may also contact this office in writing or in person at University of Minnesota Medical Center, Fairview-Riverside Campus, 2200 Riverside Avenue, Minneapolis, MN 55454. You will be given a copy of this form to keep for your records.

Statement of Consent

I have read the above information. I have asked questions and have received answers. I consent to participate in the study.

Signature of Subject_____

Signature of Investigator_____

Appendix B

HIPAA[1] AUTHORIZATION TO USE AND DISCLOSE
INDIVIDUAL HEALTH INFORMATION FOR RESEARCH PURPOSES

1. Purpose. As a research participant, I authorize Teresa J. Kimberley and the researcher's staff to use and disclose my individual health information for the purpose of conducting the research project entitled "The effect of rTMS-induced cortical inhibition on visuospatial motor skill acquisition", Human subject's code: 0802M27026.

2. Individual Health Information to be Used or Disclosed. My individual health information that may be used or disclosed to conduct this research includes: demographic information, health history regarding all current and past health concerns, family history of disease, and current medications.

3. Parties Who May Disclose My Individual Health Information. The researcher and the researcher's staff may obtain my individual health information from:

Hospitals: _____

Clinics: _____

Other Providers: _____

Health Plan: _____,

and from hospitals, clinics, health care providers and health plans that provide my health care during the study.

4. Parties Who May Receive or Use My Individual Health Information. The individual health information disclosed by parties listed in item 3 and information disclosed by me during the course of the research may be received and used by Teresa Kimberley and the researcher's staff.

5. Right to Refuse to Sign this Authorization. I do not have to sign this Authorization. If I decide not to sign the Authorization, I may not be allowed to participate in this study or receive any research related treatment that is provided through the study. However, my decision not to sign this authorization will not affect any other treatment, payment, or enrollment in health plans or eligibility for benefits.

---

[1] HIPAA is the Health Insurance Portability and Accountability Act of 1996, a federal law related to privacy of health information.

6. Right to Revoke. I can change my mind and withdraw this authorization at any time by sending a written notice to Teresa J. Kimberley, University of Minnesota, MMC 388, Minneapolis, MN 55455 to inform the researcher of my decision. If I withdraw this authorization, the researcher may only use and disclose the protected health information already collected for this research study. No further health information about me will be collected by or disclosed to the researcher for this study.

7. Potential for Re-disclosure. Once my health information is disclosed under this authorization, there is a potential that it will be re-disclosed outside this study and no longer covered by this authorization. However, the research team and the University's Institutional Review Board (the committee that reviews studies to be sure that the rights and safety of study participants are protected) are very careful to protect your privacy and limit the disclosure of identifying information about you.

> **7A.** Also, there are other laws that may require my individual health information to be disclosed for public purposes. Examples include potential disclosures if required for mandated reporting of abuse or neglect, judicial proceedings, health oversight activities and public health measures.

8. Suspension of Access. I may not be allowed to review the information collected for this study, including information recorded in my medical record, until after the study is completed. When the study is over, I will have the right to access the information again.

This authorization does not have an expiration date.

I am the research participant or personal representative authorized to act on behalf of the participant.

I have read this information, and I will receive a copy of this authorization form after it is signed.

_____
signature of research participant or research participant's personal representative

_____
date

_____
printed name of research participant or research participant's personal representative

_____
description of personal representative's authority to act on behalf of the research participant

Appendix C

Name: _____

Date: _____

Edinburgh Handedness Inventory

Indicate your preference in the use of hands
++ = The preference is so strong that you would never try to use the other hand unless absolutely forced.
+ = Your preference in use of hand.
If you are truly indifferent, put a + in both columns.
Leave blank if you have no experience in that activity.

		R	L
1	Writing		
2	Drawing		
3	Throwing		
4	Scissors		
5	Comb		
6	Toothbrush		
7	Knife (without fork)		
8	Spoon		
9	Hammer		
10	Screwdriver		
11	Tennis Racket		
12	Knife (with fork)		
13	Cricket bat (lower hand)		
14	Golf club (lower hand)		
15	Broom (upper hand)		
16	Rake (upper hand)		
17	Striking Match (match)		
18	Opening box (lid)		
19	Dealing card (card being dealt)		
20	Threading needle (needle or thread, according to which is moved.)		

Appendix D

Sleep Diary   Subject ID _____

	Night 1	Night 2
Date		
Time into Bed		
Estimated time to fall asleep		
Estimated time of waking up		
Time out of bed		
Number of times awake during the night		
Estimated amount of sleep obtained		
Naps (number, time, length)		
Alcohol or caffeinated drinks (type/amount)		
Medications used (name and time)		

Appendix E

Sleep Summary Report for SL_38_SH

Created on: 5/25/2010 2:52:19 PM

Created From File: C:\Kimberley\Gabbana\Sleep and Learning\Subjects\SL_38\SL_38_SH.dat

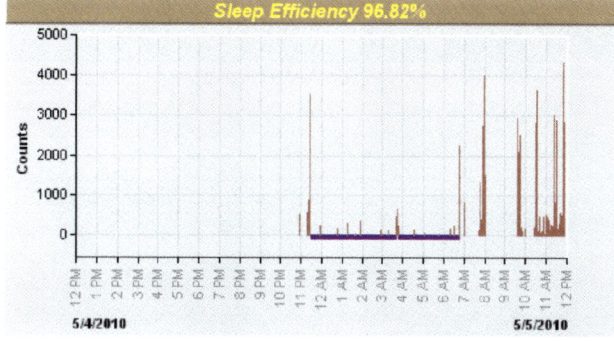

Summary for 5/4/2010

In Bed	5/4/2010 11:25 PM
Out of Bed	5/5/2010 6:45 AM
Time Asleep	7h 6m
Awakenings	3
Sleep Onset	5/4/2010 11:30:00 PM
Awake	14
Avg Awake	4m 40s
Sleep Latency	5

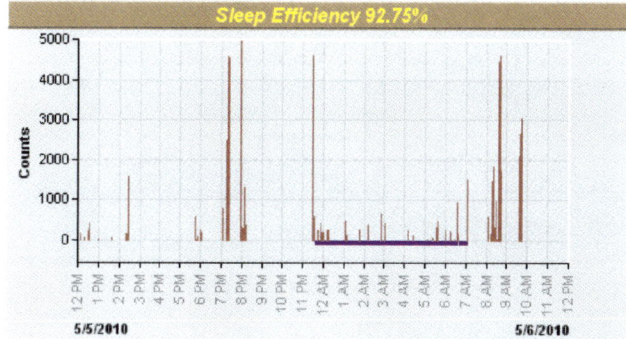

Summary for 5/5/2010

In Bed	5/5/2010 11:30 PM
Out of Bed	5/6/2010 7:05 AM
Time Asleep	7h 2m
Awakenings	15
Sleep Onset	5/5/2010 11:37:00 PM
Awake	33
Avg Awake	2m 12s
Sleep Latency	7

Sleep Data Summary

Day	In Bed	Out of Bed	Wake Minutes	Sleep Minutes	Awakenings	Efficiency	Latency
5/4/2010	11:25 PM	6:45 AM	14	426	3	96.82%	5m
5/5/2010	11:30 PM	7:05 AM	33	422	15	92.75%	7m

Appendix F

Subject ID: _____   Subject Initials: _____   Date/Time: _____

Please Rate Your Current Degree of Sleepiness:

Feeling active, vital, alert, or wide awake	1
Functioning at high levels, but not at peak; able to concentrate	2
Relaxed; awake; not at full alertness; responsive	3
A little foggy; not at peak; let down	4
Fogginess; beginning to lose interest in remaining awake; slowed down	5
Sleepiness; prefer to be lying down; fighting sleep; woozy	6
Almost in reverie; sleep onset soon; lost struggle to remain awake	7

Appendix G

Appendix. Pittsburgh Sleep Quality Index (PSQI)

Name _____ ID # _____ Date _____ Age _____

Instructions:

The following questions relate to your usual sleep habits during the past month *only*. Your answers should indicate the most accurate reply for the *majority* of days and nights in the past month. Please answer all questions.

1. During the past month, when have you usually gone to bed at night?
   USUAL BED TIME _____

2. During the past month, how long (in minutes) has it usually take you to fall asleep each night?
   NUMBER OF MINUTES _____

3. During the past month, when have you usually gotten up in the morning?
   USUAL GETTING UP TIME _____

4. During the past month, how many hours of *actual sleep* did you get at night? (This may be different than the number of hours you spend in bed.)
   HOURS OF SLEEP PER NIGHT _____

For each of the remaining questions, check the one best response. Please answer *all* questions.

5. During the past month, how often have you had trouble sleeping because you...

   (a) Cannot get to sleep within 30 minutes

Not during the past month ____	Less than once a week ____	Once or twice a week ____	Three or more times a week ____

   (b) Wake up in the middle of the night or early morning

Not during the past month ____	Less than once a week ____	Once or twice a week ____	Three or more times a week ____

   (c) Have to get up to use the bathroom

Not during the past month ____	Less than once a week ____	Once or twice a week ____	Three or more times a week ____

   (d) Cannot breathe comfortably

Not during the past month ____	Less than once a week ____	Once or twice a week ____	Three or more times a week ____

   (e) Cough or snore loudly

Not during the past month ____	Less than once a week ____	Once or twice a week ____	Three or more times a week ____

   (f) Feel too cold

Not during the past month ____	Less than once a week ____	Once or twice a week ____	Three or more times a week ____

   (g) Feel too hot

Not during the past month ____	Less than once a week ____	Once or twice a week ____	Three or more times a week ____

   (h) Had bad dreams

Not during the past month ____	Less than once a week ____	Once or twice a week ____	Three or more times a week ____

   (i) Have pain

Not during the past month ____	Less than once a week ____	Once or twice a week ____	Three or more times a week ____

(j) Other reason(s), please describe _____

How often during the past month have you had trouble sleeping because of this?
| Not during the past month _____ | Less than once a week _____ | Once or twice a week _____ | Three or more times a week _____ |

6. During the past month, how would you rate your sleep quality overall?
   Very good   _____
   Fairly good _____
   Fairly bad _____
   Very bad   _____

7. During the past month, how often have you taken medicine (prescribed or "over the counter") to help you sleep?
| Not during the past month _____ | Less than once a week _____ | Once or twice a week _____ | Three or more times a week _____ |

8. During the past month, how often have you had trouble staying awake while driving, eating meals, or engaging in social activity?
| Not during the past month _____ | Less than once a week _____ | Once or twice a week _____ | Three or more times a week _____ |

9. During the past month, how much of a problem has it been for you to keep up enough enthusiasm to get things done?
   No problem at all   _____
   Only a very slight problem _____
   Somewhat of a problem   _____
   A very big problem   _____

10. Do you have a bed partner or roommate?
    No bed partner or roommate   _____
    Partner/roommate in other room   _____
    Partner in same room, but not same bed _____
    Partner in same bed   _____

If you have a roommate or bed partner, ask him/her how often in the past month you have had...

(a) Loud snoring
| Not during the past month _____ | Less than once a week _____ | Once or twice a week _____ | Three or more times a week _____ |

(b) Long pauses between breaths while asleep
| Not during the past month _____ | Less than once a week _____ | Once or twice a week _____ | Three or more times a week _____ |

(c) Legs twitching or jerking while you sleep
| Not during the past month _____ | Less than once a week _____ | Once or twice a week _____ | Three or more times a week _____ |

(d) Episodes of disorientation or confusion during sleep
| Not during the past month _____ | Less than once a week _____ | Once or twice a week _____ | Three or more times a week _____ |

(e) Other restlessness while you sleep; please describe _____
| Not during the past month _____ | Less than once a week _____ | Once or twice a week _____ | Three or more times a week _____ |

Appendix H

Subject ID: _____   Subject Initials: _____   Date/Time: _____

Use the following scale to choose the most appropriate number for each situation:

0 = would *never* doze or sleep.
1 = *slight* chance of dozing or sleeping
2 = *moderate* chance of dozing or sleeping
3 = *high* chance of dozing or sleeping

Situation	**Chance of Dozing or Sleeping**
Sitting and reading	_____
Watching TV	_____
Sitting inactive in a public place	_____
Being a passenger in a motor vehicle for an hour or more	_____
Lying down in the afternoon	_____
Sitting and talking to someone	_____
Sitting quietly after lunch (no alcohol)	_____
Stopped for a few minutes in traffic while driving	_____
Total score	_____

Appendix I

Statistics

		rMT	aMT	@1mV
N	Valid	193	193	193
	Missing	7	7	7
Mean		44.1917	33.2694	51.8031
Std. Error of Mean		.54903	.40825	.72005
Median		44.0000	33.0000	49.0000
Mode		43.00	30.00	48.00
Std. Deviation		7.62736	5.67156	10.00326
Variance		58.177	32.167	100.065
Skewness		.342	.299	.502
Std. Error of Skewness		.175	.175	.175
Kurtosis		-.247	-.527	-.530
Std. Error of Kurtosis		.348	.348	.348
Range		36.00	24.00	40.00
Minimum		29.00	22.00	35.00
Maximum		65.00	46.00	75.00
Percentiles	2.5	31.0000	23.0000	35.8500
	97.5	60.3000	45.0000	74.1500

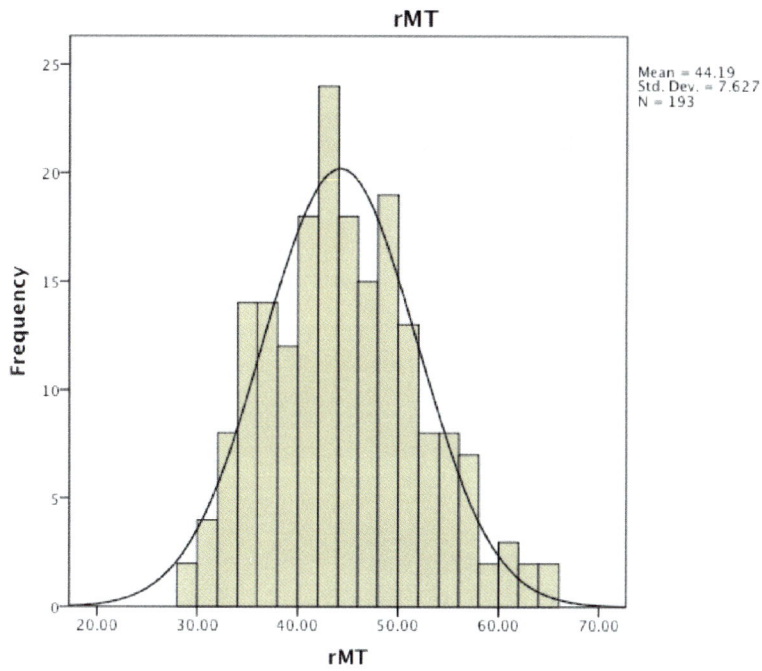

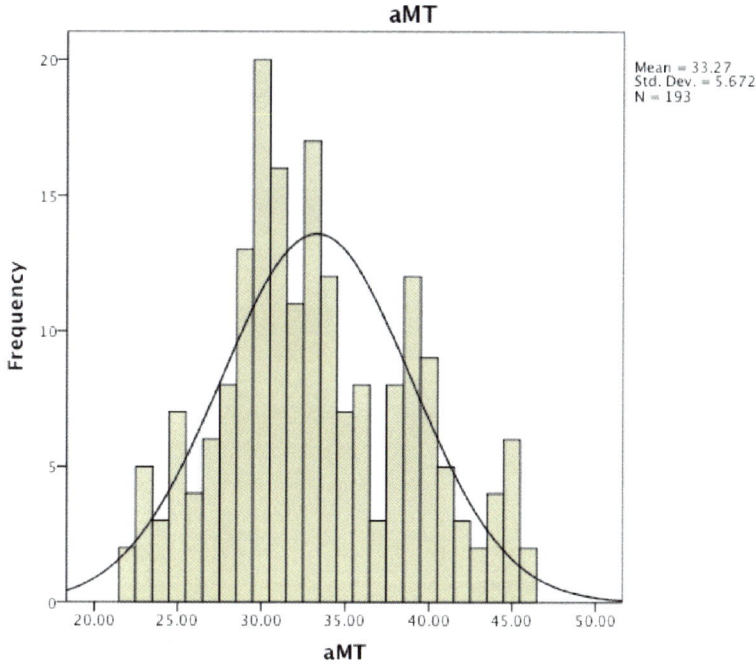

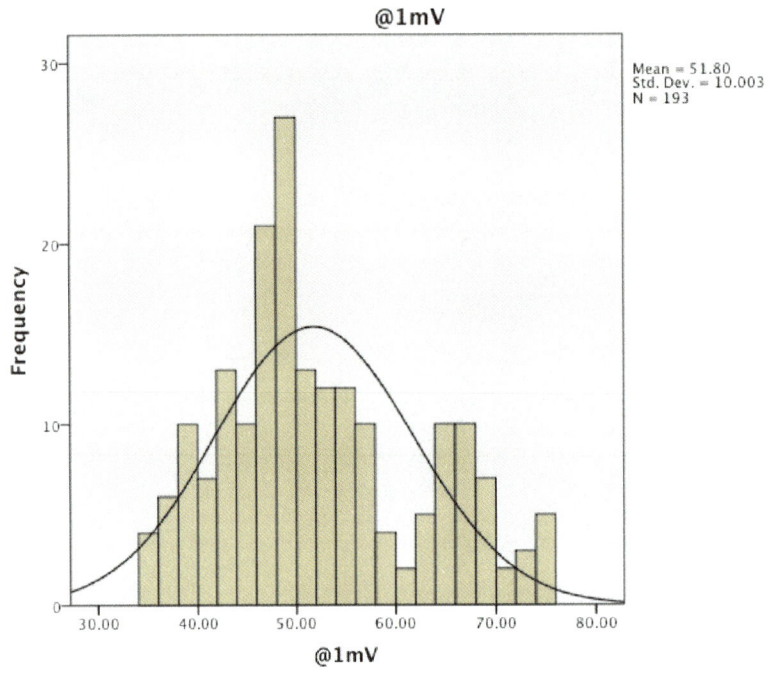

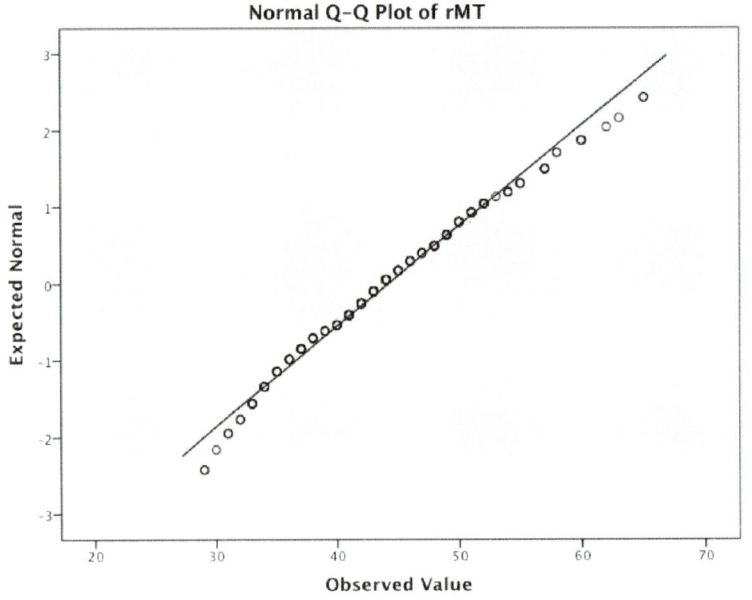

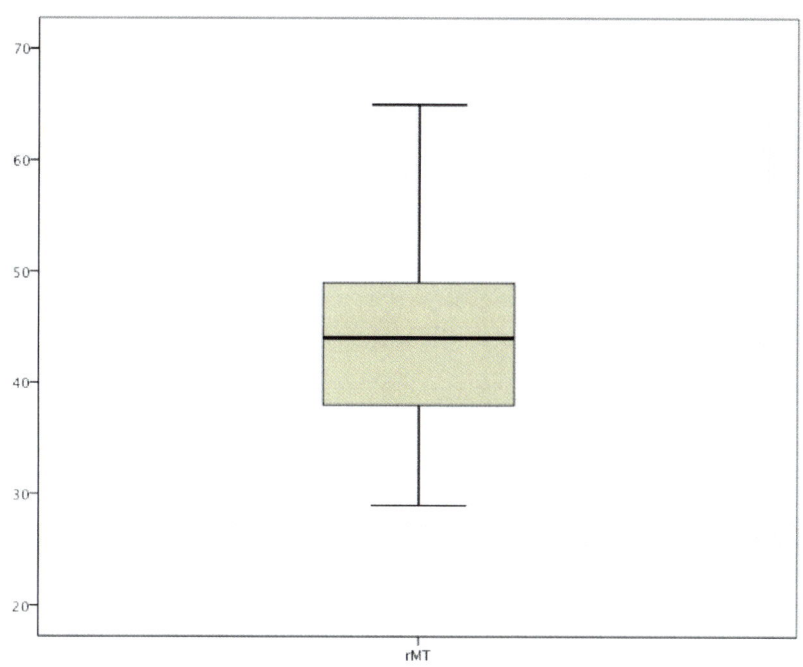

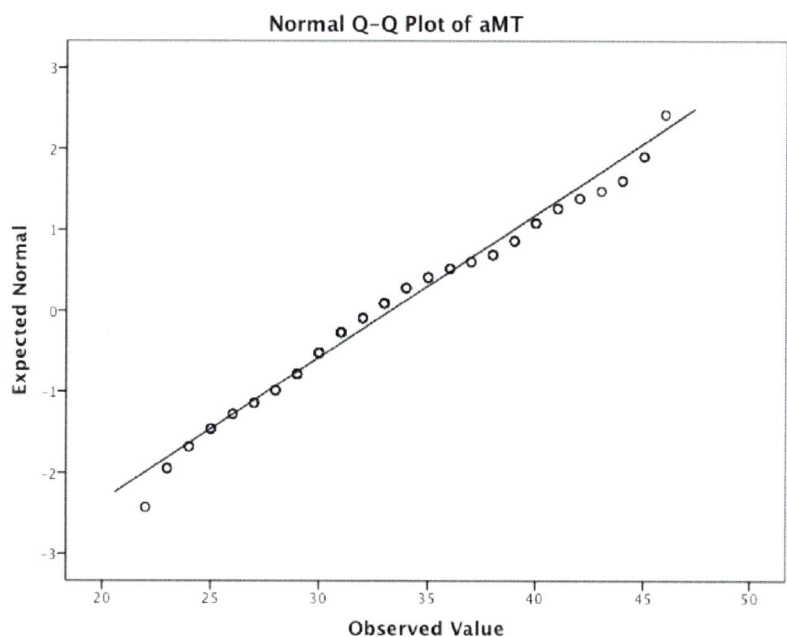

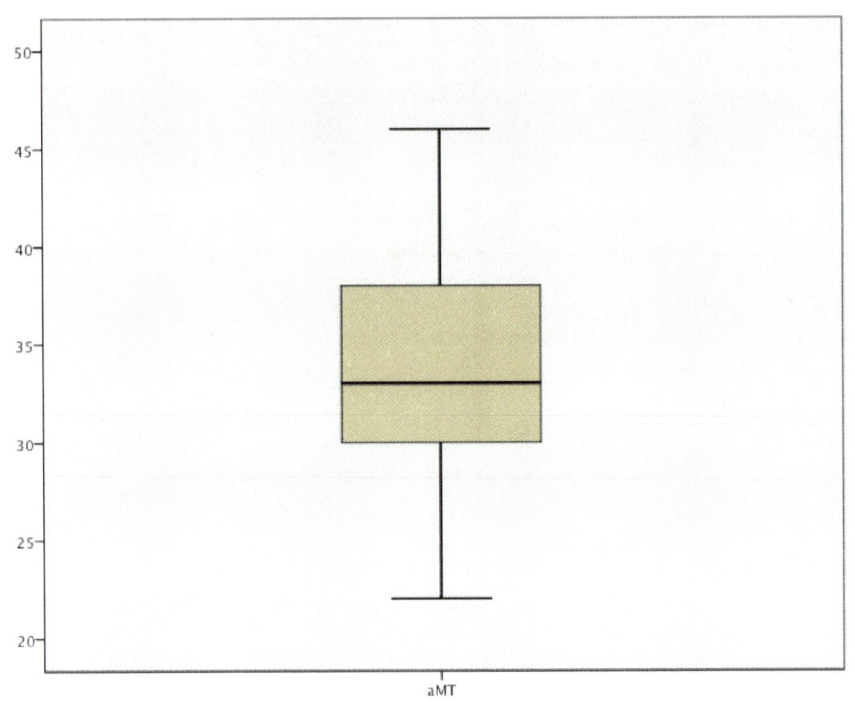

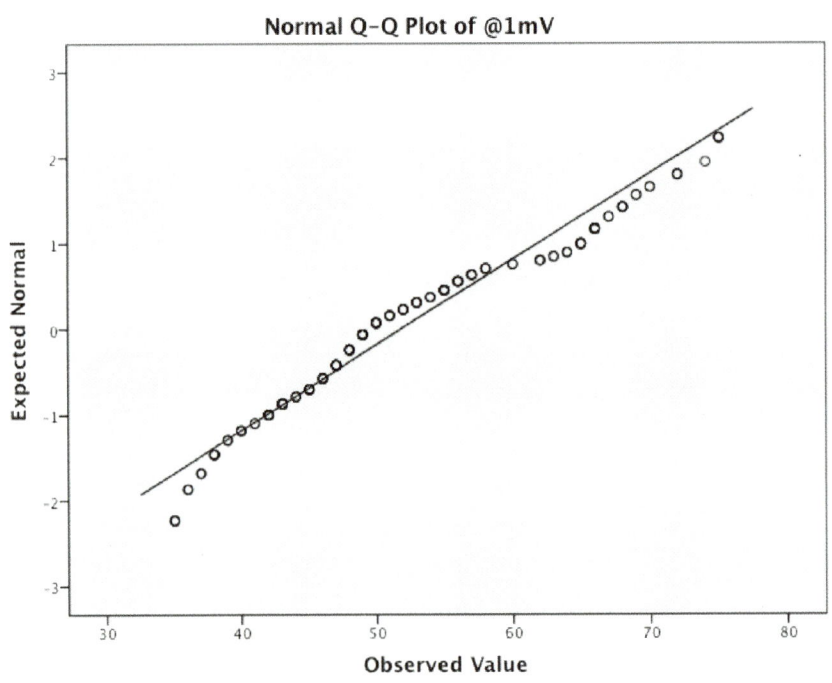

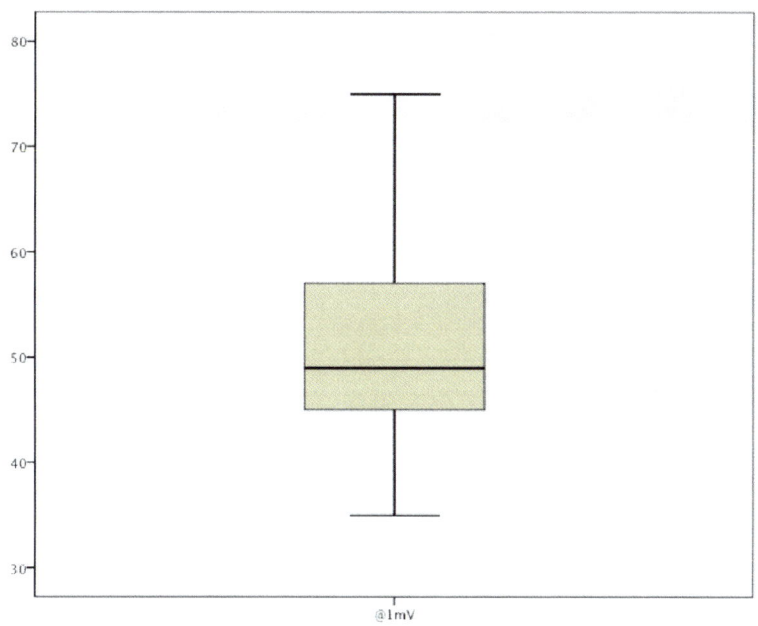

Tests of Normality

	Kolmogorov-Smirnov[a]			Shapiro-Wilk		
	Statistic	df	Sig.	Statistic	df	Sig.
rMT	.059	193	.093	.984	193	.030
aMT	.099	193	.000	.974	193	.001
@1mV	.121	193	.000	.955	193	.000

a. Lilliefors Significance Correction

Statistics[a]

		rMT	aMT	@1mV
N	Valid	85	85	85
	Missing	7	7	7
Mean		45.3765	35.1647	53.6471
Std. Error of Mean		.93275	.67131	1.25855
Median		45.0000	35.0000	51.0000
Mode		44.00	33.00	49.00
Std. Deviation		8.59952	6.18917	11.60327
Variance		73.952	38.306	134.636
Skewness		.245	-.141	.342
Std. Error of Skewness		.261	.261	.261
Kurtosis		-.580	-.704	-1.055
Std. Error of Kurtosis		.517	.517	.517
Range		36.00	24.00	40.00
Minimum		29.00	22.00	35.00
Maximum		65.00	46.00	75.00
Percentiles	2.5	31.1500	23.0000	36.0000
	97.5	64.7000	45.8500	75.0000

a. Group = 0

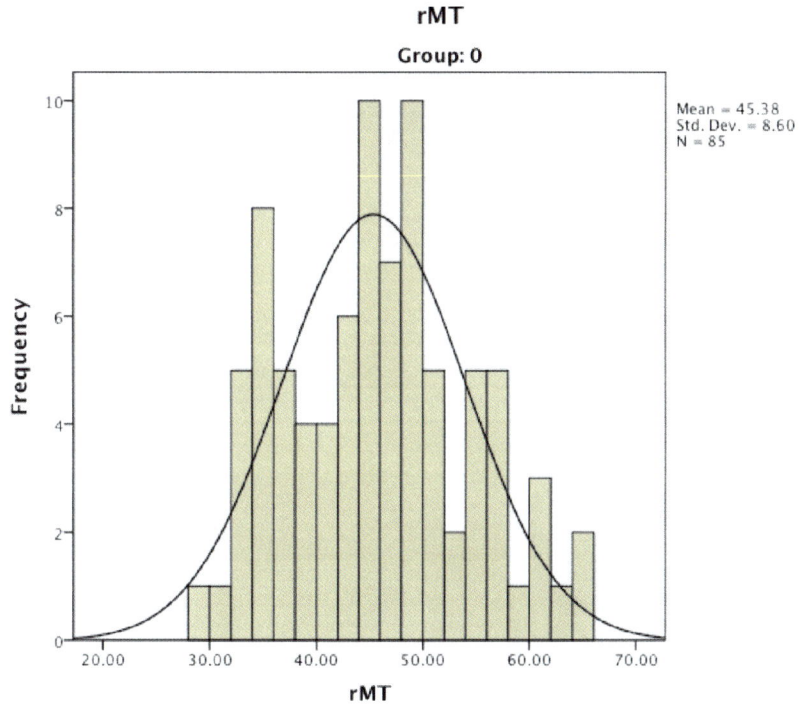

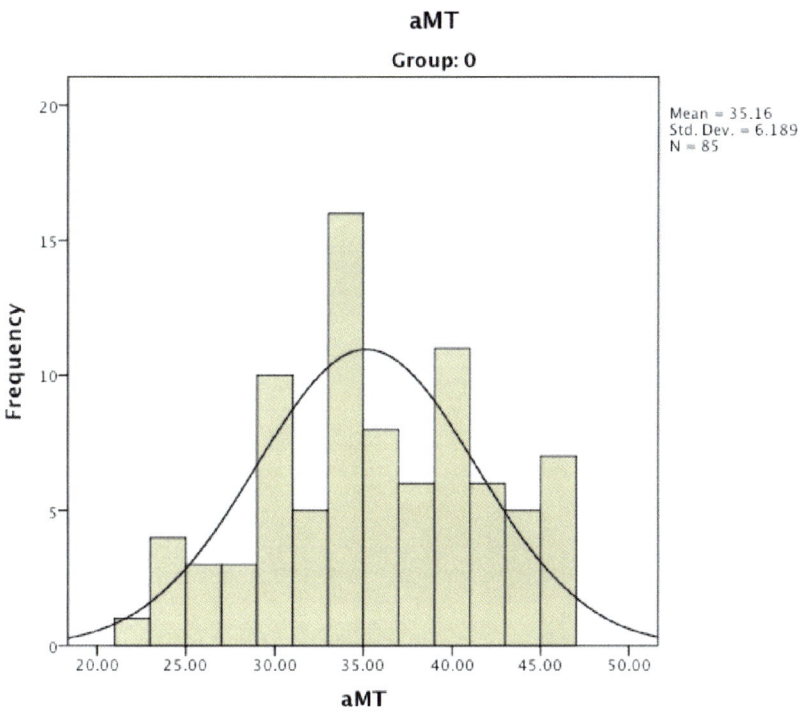

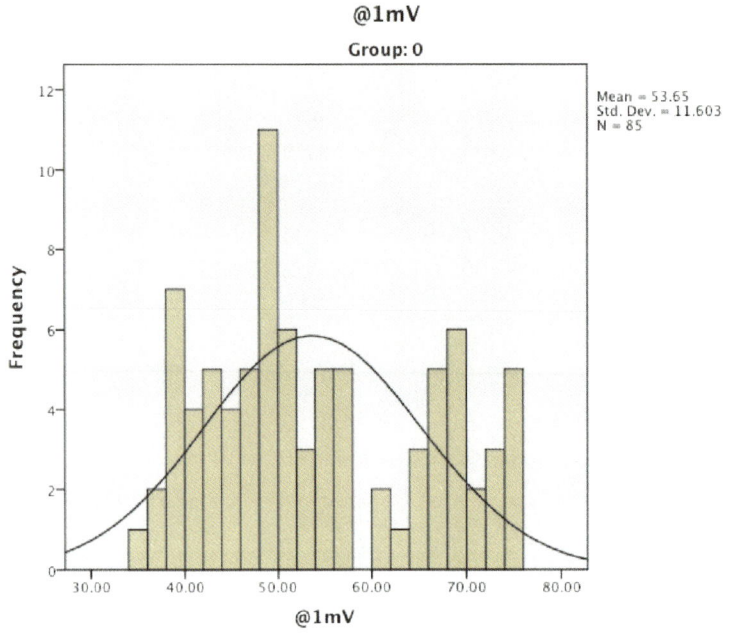

Statistics[b]

	rMT	aMT	@1mV
N Valid	80	80	80
Missing	0	0	0
Mean	43.8125	32.3500	50.7000
Std. Error of Mean	.80762	.57893	1.03061
Median	43.0000	32.0000	49.0000
Mode	41.00[a]	30.00	49.00
Std. Deviation	7.22354	5.17809	9.21803
Variance	52.180	26.813	84.972
Skewness	.006	.292	.202
Std. Error of Skewness	.269	.269	.269
Kurtosis	-.563	-.497	-.906
Std. Error of Kurtosis	.532	.532	.532
Range	33.00	23.00	33.00
Minimum	29.00	22.00	35.00
Maximum	62.00	45.00	68.00
Percentiles 2.5	30.0250	23.0000	35.0000
97.5	57.9750	43.9500	66.0000

a. Multiple modes exist. The smallest value is shown
b. Group = 1

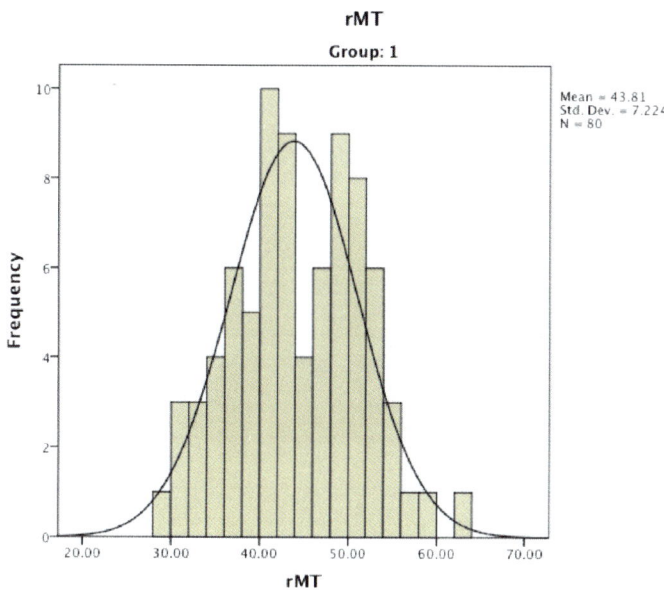

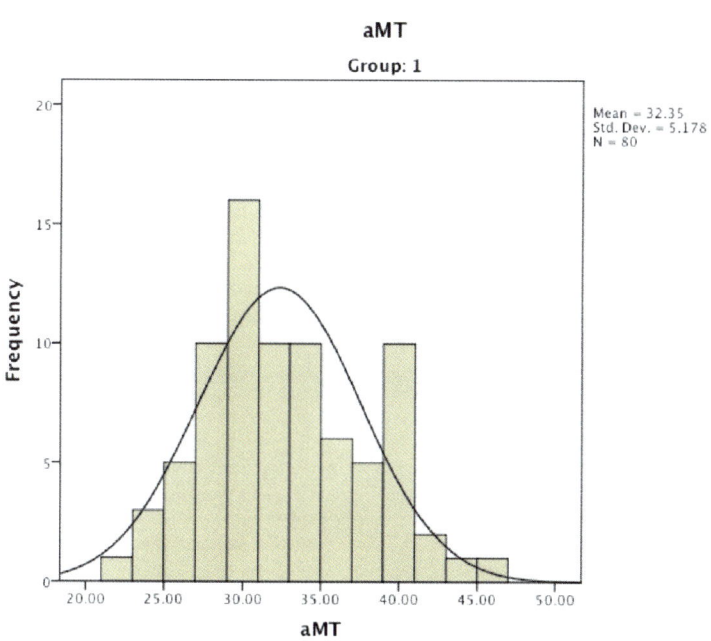

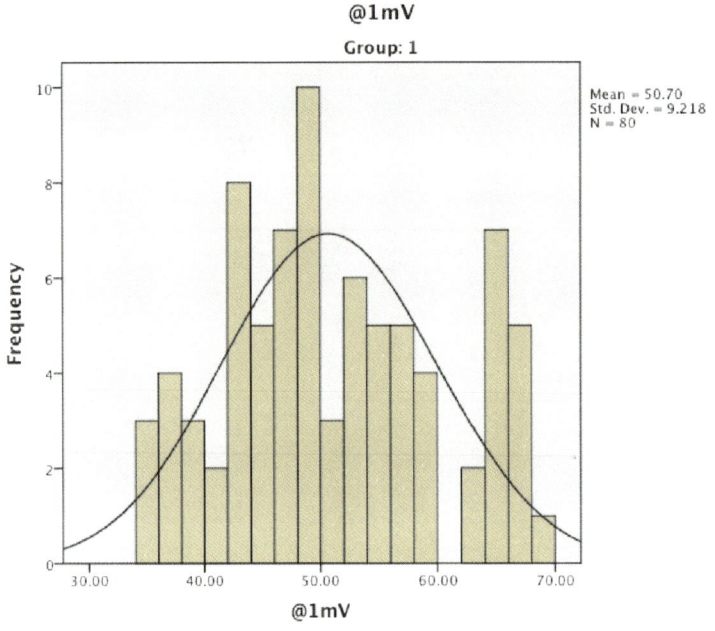

Statistics[b]

		rMT	aMT	@1mV
N	Valid	28	28	28
	Missing	0	0	0
Mean		41.6786	30.1429	49.3571
Std. Error of Mean		.83580	.50582	.91752
Median		42.0000	31.0000	48.0000
Mode		43.00	31.00	46.00[a]
Std. Deviation		4.42262	2.67657	4.85504
Variance		19.560	7.164	23.571
Skewness		1.257	-.614	1.315
Std. Error of Skewness		.441	.441	.441
Kurtosis		4.214	.749	2.546
Std. Error of Kurtosis		.858	.858	.858
Range		22.00	12.00	23.00
Minimum		35.00	24.00	40.00
Maximum		57.00	36.00	63.00
Percentiles	2.5	35.0000	24.0000	40.0000
	97.5	.	.	.

a. Multiple modes exist. The smallest value is shown

Statistics[b]

		rMT	aMT	@1mV
N	Valid	28	28	28
	Missing	0	0	0
Mean		41.6786	30.1429	49.3571
Std. Error of Mean		.83580	.50582	.91752
Median		42.0000	31.0000	48.0000
Mode		43.00	31.00	46.00[a]
Std. Deviation		4.42262	2.67657	4.85504
Variance		19.560	7.164	23.571
Skewness		1.257	-.614	1.315
Std. Error of Skewness		.441	.441	.441
Kurtosis		4.214	.749	2.546
Std. Error of Kurtosis		.858	.858	.858
Range		22.00	12.00	23.00
Minimum		35.00	24.00	40.00
Maximum		57.00	36.00	63.00
Percentiles	2.5	35.0000	24.0000	40.0000
	97.5	.	.	.

a. Multiple modes exist. The smallest value is shown
b. Group = 2

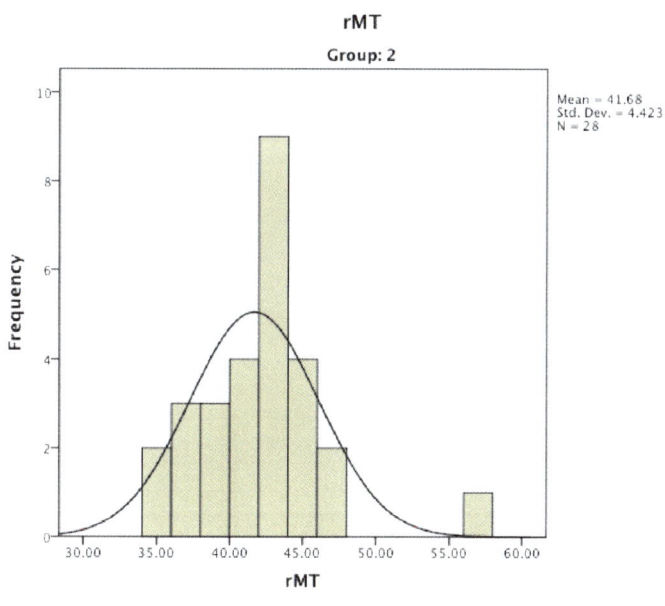

rMT
Group: 2

Mean = 41.68
Std. Dev. = 4.423
N = 28

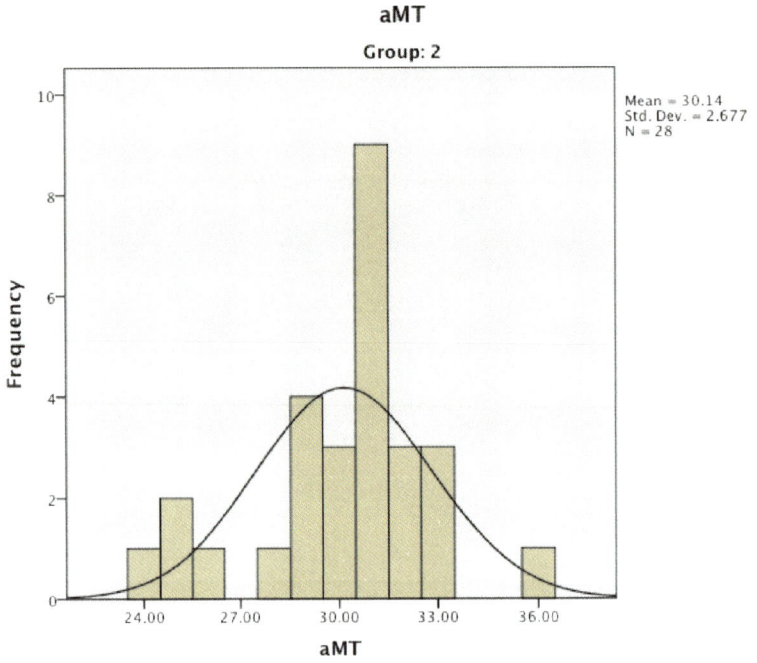
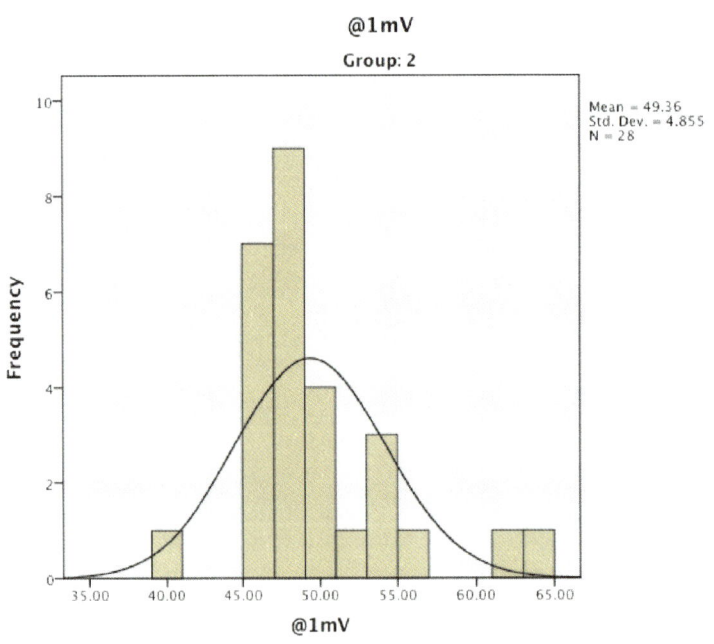

Appendix J

```
glm Accuracy_Index by Group Trial_Pol Test Polarity
 /EMMEANS = tables(Trial_Pol*Test)compare(Trial_Pol)
/EMMEANS = tables(Polarity*Test)compare(Test)
/EMMEANS = tables(Trial_Pol*Polarity)compare(Trial_Pol).
```

General Linear Model

Notes			
Output Created			17-Nov-2010 17:12:55
Comments			
Input	Data		C:\Documents and Settings\mborich\Desktop\PASW_Sleep\Tracking_full.sav
	Active Dataset		DataSet1
	Filter		Track_Train=1 (FILTER)
	Weight		<none>
	Split File		<none>
	N of Rows in Working Data File		1600
Missing Value Handling	Definition of Missing		User-defined missing values are treated as missing.
	Cases Used		Statistics are based on all cases with valid data for all variables in the model.

Syntax		glm Accuracy_Index by Group Trial_Pol Test Polarity /EMMEANS = tables(Trial_Pol*Test)compare(Trial_Pol) /EMMEANS = tables(Polarity*Test)compare(Test) /EMMEANS = tables(Trial_Pol*Polarity)compare(Trial_Pol).
Resources	Processor Time	00:00:00.297
	Elapsed Time	00:00:00.313

```
[DataSet1] C:\Documents and Settings\mborich\Desktop\PASW_Sleep\Tracking_full.sav
```

Between-Subjects Factors

		N
Group	0	790
	1	780
Trial_Pol	1	314
	2	314
	3	314
	4	314
	5	314
Test	1	390
	2	400
	3	400
	4	380
Polarity	0	785
	1	785

Tests of Between-Subjects Effects

Dependent Variable:Accuracy_Index

Source	Type III Sum of Squares	df	Mean Square	F	Sig.
Corrected Model	20.634[a]	79	.261	10.218	.000
Intercept	501.748	1	501.748	19629.399	.000
Group	.030	1	.030	1.191	.275
Trial_Pol	2.143	4	.536	20.957	.000
Test	7.342	3	2.447	95.744	.000
Polarity	5.813	1	5.813	227.410	.000
Group * Trial_Pol	.037	4	.009	.360	.837
Group * Test	.028	3	.009	.370	.774
Group * Polarity	.022	1	.022	.860	.354
Trial_Pol * Test	2.518	12	.210	8.208	.000
Trial_Pol * Polarity	.525	4	.131	5.131	.000
Test * Polarity	.717	3	.239	9.345	.000
Group * Trial_Pol * Test	.208	12	.017	.678	.774
Group * Trial_Pol * Polarity	.149	4	.037	1.454	.214
Group * Test * Polarity	.062	3	.021	.811	.487
Trial_Pol * Test * Polarity	.819	12	.068	2.671	.001
Group * Trial_Pol * Test * Polarity	.314	12	.026	1.024	.424
Error	38.086	1490	.026		
Total	560.619	1570			
Corrected Total	58.720	1569			

a. R Squared = .351 (Adjusted R Squared = .317)

Estimated Marginal Means

1. Trial_Pol * Test

Estimates

Dependent Variable: Accuracy_Index

Trial_Pol	Test	Mean	Std. Error	95% Confidence Interval	
				Lower Bound	Upper Bound
1	1	.262	.018	.227	.298
	2	.559	.018	.524	.594
	3	.562	.018	.527	.597
	4	.601	.018	.565	.637
2	1	.432	.018	.397	.468
	2	.576	.018	.540	.611
	3	.606	.018	.571	.641
	4	.625	.018	.589	.661
3	1	.479	.018	.444	.515
	2	.579	.018	.544	.614
	3	.631	.018	.596	.666
	4	.647	.018	.611	.683
4	1	.557	.018	.521	.592
	2	.580	.018	.545	.615
	3	.614	.018	.579	.649
	4	.635	.018	.599	.671
5	1	.532	.018	.496	.567
	2	.559	.018	.523	.594
	3	.631	.018	.596	.666

Estimates

Dependent Variable: Accuracy_Index

Trial_Pol	Test	Mean	Std. Error	95% Confidence Interval	
				Lower Bound	Upper Bound
1	1	.262	.018	.227	.298
	2	.559	.018	.524	.594
	3	.562	.018	.527	.597
	4	.601	.018	.565	.637
2	1	.432	.018	.397	.468
	2	.576	.018	.540	.611
	3	.606	.018	.571	.641
	4	.625	.018	.589	.661
3	1	.479	.018	.444	.515
	2	.579	.018	.544	.614
	3	.631	.018	.596	.666
	4	.647	.018	.611	.683
4	1	.557	.018	.521	.592
	2	.580	.018	.545	.615
	3	.614	.018	.579	.649
	4	.635	.018	.599	.671
	1	.532	.018	.496	.567
	2	.559	.018	.523	.594
	3	.631	.018	.596	.666
	4	.643	.018	.607	.679

Pairwise Comparisons

Dependent Variable:Accuracy_Index

Test	(I) Trial_Pol	(J) Trial_Pol	Mean Difference (I-J)	Std. Error	Sig.[a]	95% Confidence Interval for Difference[a]	
						Lower Bound	Upper Bound
1	1	2	-.170*	.026	.000	-.220	-.120
		3	-.217*	.026	.000	-.267	-.167
		4	-.295*	.026	.000	-.345	-.244
		5	-.269*	.026	.000	-.319	-.219
	2	1	.170*	.026	.000	.120	.220
		3	-.047	.026	.067	-.097	.003
		4	-.125*	.026	.000	-.175	-.074
		5	-.099*	.026	.000	-.150	-.049
	3	1	.217*	.026	.000	.167	.267
		2	.047	.026	.067	-.003	.097
		4	-.078*	.026	.002	-.128	-.027
		5	-.052*	.026	.041	-.103	-.002
	4	1	.295*	.026	.000	.244	.345
		2	.125*	.026	.000	.074	.175
		3	.078*	.026	.002	.027	.128
		5	.025	.026	.324	-.025	.076
	5	1	.269*	.026	.000	.219	.319
		2	.099*	.026	.000	.049	.150
		3	.052*	.026	.041	.002	.103
		4	-.025	.026	.324	-.076	.025
2	1	2	-.016	.025	.515	-.066	.033
		3	-.020	.025	.433	-.069	.030
		4	-.021	.025	.400	-.071	.028

			5	.001	.025	.982	-.049	.050
		2	1	.016	.025	.515	-.033	.066
			3	-.003	.025	.895	-.053	.046
			4	-.005	.025	.849	-.054	.045
			5	.017	.025	.501	-.033	.067
		3	1	.020	.025	.433	-.030	.069
			2	.003	.025	.895	-.046	.053
			4	-.001	.025	.954	-.051	.048
			5	.020	.025	.420	-.029	.070
		4	1	.021	.025	.400	-.028	.071
			2	.005	.025	.849	-.045	.054
			3	.001	.025	.954	-.048	.051
			5	.022	.025	.388	-.028	.071
		5	1	-.001	.025	.982	-.050	.049
			2	-.017	.025	.501	-.067	.033
			3	-.020	.025	.420	-.070	.029
			4	-.022	.025	.388	-.071	.028
3	1		2	-.044	.025	.081	-.094	.005
			3	-.069*	.025	.006	-.119	-.020
			4	-.052*	.025	.039	-.102	-.003
			5	-.069*	.025	.006	-.119	-.019
		2	1	.044	.025	.081	-.005	.094
			3	-.025	.025	.317	-.075	.024
			4	-.008	.025	.750	-.058	.042
			5	-.025	.025	.323	-.075	.025
		3	1	.069*	.025	.006	.020	.119
			2	.025	.025	.317	-.024	.075

			4	.017	.025	.495	-.032	.067
			5	.000	.025	.989	-.049	.050
		4	1	.052*	.025	.039	.003	.102
			2	.008	.025	.750	-.042	.058
			3	-.017	.025	.495	-.067	.032
			5	-.017	.025	.503	-.067	.033
		5	1	.069*	.025	.006	.019	.119
			2	.025	.025	.323	-.025	.075
			3	.000	.025	.989	-.050	.049
			4	.017	.025	.503	-.033	.067
4	1	2		-.024	.026	.357	-.075	.027
		3		-.046	.026	.074	-.097	.005
		4		-.034	.026	.184	-.085	.016
		5		-.042	.026	.104	-.093	.009
	2	1		.024	.026	.357	-.027	.075
		3		-.022	.026	.387	-.073	.028
		4		-.011	.026	.683	-.061	.040
		5		-.018	.026	.480	-.069	.033
	3	1		.046	.026	.074	-.005	.097
		2		.022	.026	.387	-.028	.073
		4		.012	.026	.648	-.039	.063
		5		.004	.026	.875	-.047	.055
	4	1		.034	.026	.184	-.016	.085
		2		.011	.026	.683	-.040	.061
		3		-.012	.026	.648	-.063	.039
		5		-.008	.026	.766	-.059	.043

	5	1	.042	.026	.104	-.009	.093
		2	.018	.026	.480	-.033	.069
		3	-.004	.026	.875	-.055	.047
		4	.008	.026	.766	-.043	.059

Based on estimated marginal means

*. The mean difference is significant at the .050 level.

a. Adjustment for multiple comparisons: Least Significant Difference (equivalent to no adjustments).

Univariate Tests

Dependent Variable:Accuracy_Index

Test		Sum of Squares	df	Mean Square	F	Sig.
1	Contrast	4.242	4	1.061	41.494	.000
	Error	38.086	1490	.026		
2	Contrast	.037	4	.009	.365	.833
	Error	38.086	1490	.026		
3	Contrast	.259	4	.065	2.530	.039
	Error	38.086	1490	.026		
4	Contrast	.104	4	.026	1.019	.396
	Error	38.086	1490	.026		

Each F tests the simple effects of Trial_Pol within each level combination of the other effects shown. These tests are based on the linearly independent pairwise comparisons among the estimated marginal means.

2. Polarity * Test

Estimates

Dependent Variable:Accuracy_Index

Polarity	Test	Mean	Std. Error	95% Confidence Interval	
				Lower Bound	Upper Bound

0	1	.547	.011	.525	.569
	2	.634	.011	.612	.656
	3	.655	.011	.633	.677
	4	.669	.012	.647	.692
1	1	.358	.011	.335	.380
	2	.507	.011	.484	.529
	3	.563	.011	.541	.585
	4	.591	.012	.568	.614

Pairwise Comparisons

Dependent Variable:Accuracy_Index

Polarity	(I) Test	(J) Test	Mean Difference (I-J)	Std. Error	Sig.[a]	95% Confidence Interval for Difference[a]	
						Lower Bound	Upper Bound
0	1	2	-.087*	.016	.000	-.119	-.056
		3	-.108*	.016	.000	-.139	-.076
		4	-.122*	.016	.000	-.154	-.090
	2	1	.087*	.016	.000	.056	.119
		3	-.020	.016	.200	-.052	.011
		4	-.035*	.016	.030	-.067	-.003
	3	1	.108*	.016	.000	.076	.139
		2	.020	.016	.200	-.011	.052
		4	-.015	.016	.366	-.046	.017
	4	1	.122*	.016	.000	.090	.154
		2	.035*	.016	.030	.003	.067
		3	.015	.016	.366	-.017	.046

1	1	2	-.149*	.016	.000	-.180	-.117
		3	-.205*	.016	.000	-.237	-.174
		4	-.233*	.016	.000	-.265	-.201
	2	1	.149*	.016	.000	.117	.180
		3	-.056*	.016	.000	-.088	-.025
		4	-.085*	.016	.000	-.116	-.053
	3	1	.205*	.016	.000	.174	.237
		2	.056*	.016	.000	.025	.088
		4	-.028	.016	.080	-.060	.003
	4	1	.233*	.016	.000	.201	.265
		2	.085*	.016	.000	.053	.116
		3	.028	.016	.080	-.003	.060

Based on estimated marginal means

*. The mean difference is significant at the .050 level.

a. Adjustment for multiple comparisons: Least Significant Difference (equivalent to no adjustments).

Univariate Tests

Dependent Variable:Accuracy_Index

Polarity		Sum of Squares	df	Mean Square	F	Sig.
0	Contrast	1.753	3	.584	22.855	.000
	Error	38.086	1490	.026		
1	Contrast	6.306	3	2.102	82.234	.000
	Error	38.086	1490	.026		

Each F tests the simple effects of Test within each level combination of the other effects shown. These tests are based on the linearly independent pairwise comparisons among the estimated marginal means.

3. Trial_Pol * Polarity

Estimates

Dependent Variable:Accuracy_Index

Trial_Pol	Polarity	Mean	Std. Error	95% Confidence Interval	
				Lower Bound	Upper Bound
1	0	.590	.013	.564	.615
	1	.403	.013	.378	.428
2	0	.627	.013	.602	.652
	1	.492	.013	.467	.517
3	0	.636	.013	.611	.661
	1	.532	.013	.507	.557
4	0	.640	.013	.615	.665
	1	.554	.013	.529	.579
5	0	.639	.013	.614	.664
	1	.543	.013	.518	.568

Pairwise Comparisons

Dependent Variable:Accuracy_Index

Polarity	(I) Trial_Pol	(J) Trial_Pol	Mean Difference (I-J)	Std. Error	Sig.[a]	95% Confidence Interval for Difference[a]	
						Lower Bound	Upper Bound
0	1	2	-.038*	.018	.036	-.073	-.002
		3	-.047*	.018	.010	-.082	-.011
		4	-.050*	.018	.006	-.086	-.015
		5	-.050*	.018	.006	-.085	-.014
	2	1	.038*	.018	.036	.002	.073
		3	-.009	.018	.631	-.044	.027

			4	-.012	.018	.495	-.048	.023
			5	-.012	.018	.515	-.047	.024
		3	1	.047*	.018	.010	.011	.082
			2	.009	.018	.631	-.027	.044
			4	-.004	.018	.840	-.039	.032
			5	-.003	.018	.865	-.038	.032
		4	1	.050*	.018	.006	.015	.086
			2	.012	.018	.495	-.023	.048
			3	.004	.018	.840	-.032	.039
			5	.001	.018	.975	-.035	.036
		5	1	.050*	.018	.006	.014	.085
			2	.012	.018	.515	-.024	.047
			3	.003	.018	.865	-.032	.038
			4	-.001	.018	.975	-.036	.035
1	1		2	-.089*	.018	.000	-.125	-.054
			3	-.130*	.018	.000	-.165	-.094
			4	-.151*	.018	.000	-.186	-.116
			5	-.140*	.018	.000	-.176	-.105
	2		1	.089*	.018	.000	.054	.125
			3	-.040*	.018	.025	-.076	-.005
			4	-.062*	.018	.001	-.097	-.026
			5	-.051*	.018	.005	-.087	-.016
	3		1	.130*	.018	.000	.094	.165
			2	.040*	.018	.025	.005	.076
			4	-.021	.018	.236	-.057	.014

			-.011	.018	.552	-.046	.025
	5						
	4	1	.151*	.018	.000	.116	.186
		2	.062*	.018	.001	.026	.097
		3	.021	.018	.236	-.014	.057
		5	.011	.018	.555	-.025	.046
	5	1	.140*	.018	.000	.105	.176
		2	.051*	.018	.005	.016	.087
		3	.011	.018	.552	-.025	.046
		4	-.011	.018	.555	-.046	.025

Based on estimated marginal means

*. The mean difference is significant at the .050 level.

a. Adjustment for multiple comparisons: Least Significant Difference (equivalent to no adjustments).

Univariate Tests

Dependent Variable:Accuracy_Index

Polarity		Sum of Squares	df	Mean Square	F	Sig.
0	Contrast	.281	4	.070	2.751	.027
	Error	38.086	1490	.026		
1	Contrast	2.386	4	.597	23.337	.000
	Error	38.086	1490	.026		

Each F tests the simple effects of Trial_Pol within each level combination of the other effects shown. These tests are based on the linearly independent pairwise comparisons among the estimated marginal means.

Appendix K

General Linear Model

Notes		
Output Created		11-Nov-2010 15:56:17
Comments		
Input	Active Dataset	DataSet8
	Filter	Track_Train=1 (FILTER)
	Weight	<none>
	Split File	<none>
	N of Rows in Working Data File	40
Missing Value Handling	Definition of Missing	User-defined missing values are treated as missing.
	Cases Used	Statistics are based on all cases with valid data for all variables in the model.

Syntax		GLM AI_comp.1.00 AI_comp.2.00 AI_comp.3.00 AI_comp.4.00 BY Group /WSFACTOR=Test 4 Polynomial /METHOD=SSTYPE(3) /PLOT=PROFILE(Test*Group) /EMMEANS=TABLES(Group) COMPARE ADJ(LSD) /EMMEANS=TABLES(Test) COMPARE ADJ(LSD) /EMMEANS=TABLES(Group*Test) /PRINT=DESCRIPTIVE ETASQ OPOWER HOMOGENEITY /CRITERIA=ALPHA(.05) /WSDESIGN=Test /DESIGN=Group.
Resources	Processor Time	00:00:00.203
	Elapsed Time	00:00:00.203

[DataSet8] C:\Documents and Settings\mborich\Desktop\PASW_Sleep\Tracking_mean_notrial1.sav

Within-Subjects Factors

Measure:MEASURE_1

Test	Dependent Variable
1	AI_comp.1.00
2	AI_comp.2.00

| 3 | Al_comp.3.00 |
| 4 | Al_comp.4.00 |

Between-Subjects Factors

		N
Group	.00	19
	1.00	18

Descriptive Statistics

	Group	Mean	Std. Deviation	N
Al_comp.1.00	.00	.5727	.12976	19
	1.00	.5785	.08447	18
	Total	.5755	.10862	37
Al_comp.2.00	.00	.6247	.09770	19
	1.00	.6390	.05627	18

	Total	.6316	.07950	37
AI_comp.3.00	.00	.6641	.07903	19
	1.00	.6601	.06178	18
	Total	.6622	.07021	37
AI_comp.4.00	.00	.6617	.08885	19
	1.00	.6815	.04902	18
	Total	.6714	.07199	37

Box's Test of Equality of Covariance Matrices[a]

Box's M	16.976
F	1.486
df1	10
df2	5813.608

Sig.	.138

Tests the null hypothesis that the observed covariance matrices of the dependent variables are equal across groups.

a. Design: Intercept + Group

Within Subjects Design: Test

Multivariate Tests[c]

Effect		Value	F	Hypothesis df	Error df	Sig.	Partial Eta Squared	Noncent. Parameter	Observed Power[b]
Test	Pillai's Trace	.658	21.128[a]	3.000	33.000	.000	.658	63.384	1.000
	Wilks' Lambda	.342	21.128[a]	3.000	33.000	.000	.658	63.384	1.000
	Hotelling's Trace	1.921	21.128[a]	3.000	33.000	.000	.658	63.384	1.000
	Roy's Largest Root	1.921	21.128[a]	3.000	33.000	.000	.658	63.384	1.000
Test * Group	Pillai's Trace	.079	.945[a]	3.000	33.000	.430	.079	2.836	.235
	Wilks' Lambda	.921	.945[a]	3.000	33.000	.430	.079	2.836	.235
	Hotelling's Trace	.086	.945[a]	3.000	33.000	.430	.079	2.836	.235
	Roy's Largest Root	.086	.945[a]	3.000	33.000	.430	.079	2.836	.235

a. Exact statistic

b. Computed using alpha = .05

Multivariate Tests[c]

Effect		Value	F	Hypothesis df	Error df	Sig.	Partial Eta Squared	Noncent. Parameter	Observed Power[b]
Test	Pillai's Trace	.658	21.128[a]	3.000	33.000	.000	.658	63.384	1.000
	Wilks' Lambda	.342	21.128[a]	3.000	33.000	.000	.658	63.384	1.000
	Hotelling's Trace	1.921	21.128[a]	3.000	33.000	.000	.658	63.384	1.000
	Roy's Largest Root	1.921	21.128[a]	3.000	33.000	.000	.658	63.384	1.000
Test * Group	Pillai's Trace	.079	.945[a]	3.000	33.000	.430	.079	2.836	.235
	Wilks' Lambda	.921	.945[a]	3.000	33.000	.430	.079	2.836	.235
	Hotelling's Trace	.086	.945[a]	3.000	33.000	.430	.079	2.836	.235
	Roy's Largest Root	.086	.945[a]	3.000	33.000	.430	.079	2.836	.235

a. Exact statistic

b. Computed using alpha = .05

c. Design: Intercept + Group
 Within Subjects Design: Test

Mauchly's Test of Sphericity[b]

Measure:MEASURE_1

Within Subjects Effect	Mauchly's W	Approx. Chi-Square	df	Sig.	Epsilon[a]		
					Greenhouse-Geisser	Huynh-Feldt	Lower-bound
Test	.546	20.387	5	.001	.713	.783	.333

Tests the null hypothesis that the error covariance matrix of the orthonormalized transformed dependent variables is proportional to an identity matrix.

a. May be used to adjust the degrees of freedom for the averaged tests of significance. Corrected tests are displayed in the Tests of Within-Subjects Effects table.

b. Design: Intercept + Group
 Within Subjects Design: Test

Tests of Within-Subjects Effects

Measure:MEASURE_1

Source		Type III Sum of Squares	df	Mean Square	F	Sig.	Partial Eta Squared	Noncent. Parameter	Observed Power[a]
Test	Sphericity Assumed	.208	3	.069	30.916	.000	.469	92.748	1.000
	Greenhouse-Geisser	.208	2.139	.097	30.916	.000	.469	66.140	1.000
	Huynh-Feldt	.208	2.348	.088	30.916	.000	.469	72.590	1.000
	Lower-bound	.208	1.000	.208	30.916	.000	.469	30.916	1.000
Test * Group	Sphericity Assumed	.003	3	.001	.448	.719	.013	1.343	.137
	Greenhouse-Geisser	.003	2.139	.001	.448	.654	.013	.958	.123
	Huynh-Feldt	.003	2.348	.001	.448	.672	.013	1.051	.126
	Lower-bound	.003	1.000	.003	.448	.508	.013	.448	.100
Error(Test)	Sphericity Assumed	.235	105	.002					
	Greenhouse-Geisser	.235	74.877	.003					
	Huynh-Feldt	.235	82.179	.003					
	Lower-bound	.235	35.000	.007					

Tests of Within-Subjects Effects

Measure:MEASURE_1

Source		Type III Sum of Squares	df	Mean Square	F	Sig.	Partial Eta Squared	Noncent. Parameter	Observed Power[a]
Test	Sphericity Assumed	.208	3	.069	30.916	.000	.469	92.748	1.000
	Greenhouse-Geisser	.208	2.139	.097	30.916	.000	.469	66.140	1.000
	Huynh-Feldt	.208	2.348	.088	30.916	.000	.469	72.590	1.000
	Lower-bound	.208	1.000	.208	30.916	.000	.469	30.916	1.000
Test * Group	Sphericity Assumed	.003	3	.001	.448	.719	.013	1.343	.137
	Greenhouse-Geisser	.003	2.139	.001	.448	.654	.013	.958	.123
	Huynh-Feldt	.003	2.348	.001	.448	.672	.013	1.051	.126
	Lower-bound	.003	1.000	.003	.448	.508	.013	.448	.100
Error(Test)	Sphericity Assumed	.235	105	.002					
	Greenhouse-Geisser	.235	74.877	.003					
	Huynh-Feldt	.235	82.179	.003					
	Lower-bound	.235	35.000	.007					

a. Computed using alpha = .05

Tests of Within-Subjects Contrasts

Measure:MEASURE_1

Source	Test	Type III Sum of Squares	df	Mean Square	F	Sig.	Partial Eta Squared	Noncent. Parameter	Observed Power[a]
Test	Linear	.187	1	.187	63.888	.000	.646	63.888	1.000
	Quadratic	.020	1	.020	8.829	.005	.201	8.829	.824
	Cubic	5.029E-5	1	5.029E-5	.034	.856	.001	.034	.054
Test * Group	Linear	.000	1	.000	.090	.766	.003	.090	.060
	Quadratic	.001	1	.001	.239	.628	.007	.239	.076
	Cubic	.002	1	.002	1.469	.234	.040	1.469	.218
Error(Test)	Linear	.103	35	.003					
	Quadratic	.080	35	.002					
	Cubic	.052	35	.001					

a. Computed using alpha = .05

Levene's Test of Equality of Error Variances[a]

	F	df1	df2	Sig.
AI_comp.1.00	2.106	1	35	.156
AI_comp.2.00	2.048	1	35	.161
AI_comp.3.00	.460	1	35	.502
AI_comp.4.00	2.043	1	35	.162

Tests the null hypothesis that the error variance of the dependent variable is equal across groups.

a. Design: Intercept + Group
Within Subjects Design: Test

Tests of Between-Subjects Effects

Measure:MEASURE_1

Transformed Variable:Average

Source	Type III Sum of Squares	df	Mean Square	F	Sig.	Partial Eta Squared	Noncent. Parameter	Observed Power[a]
Intercept	59.688	1	59.688	2694.661	.000	.987	2694.661	1.000
Group	.003	1	.003	.134	.716	.004	.134	.065
Error	.775	35	.022					

a. Computed using alpha = .05

Estimated Marginal Means

1. Group

Estimates

Measure:MEASURE_1

Group	Mean	Std. Error	95% Confidence Interval	
			Lower Bound	Upper Bound
.00	.631	.017	.596	.665
1.00	.640	.018	.604	.675

Pairwise Comparisons

Measure:MEASURE_1

(I) Group	(J) Group	Mean Difference (I-J)	Std. Error	Sig.[a]	95% Confidence Interval for Difference[a]	
					Lower Bound	Upper Bound
.00	1.00	-.009	.024	.716	-.059	.041
1.00	.00	.009	.024	.716	-.041	.059

Based on estimated marginal means

a. Adjustment for multiple comparisons: Least Significant Difference (equivalent to no adjustments).

Univariate Tests

Measure:MEASURE_1

	Sum of Squares	df	Mean Square	F	Sig.	Partial Eta Squared	Noncent. Parameter	Observed Power[a]
Contrast	.001	1	.001	.134	.716	.004	.134	.065
Error	.194	35	.006					

The F tests the effect of Group. This test is based on the linearly independent pairwise comparisons among the estimated marginal means.

a. Computed using alpha = .05

2. Test

Estimates

Measure:MEASURE_1

Test	Mean	Std. Error	95% Confidence Interval	
			Lower Bound	Upper Bound
1	.576	.018	.539	.612
2	.632	.013	.605	.659

3	.662	.012	.638	.686
4	.672	.012	.647	.696

Pairwise Comparisons

Measure:MEASURE_1

(I) Test	(J) Test	Mean Difference (I-J)	Std. Error	Sig.[a]	95% Confidence Interval for Difference[a]	
					Lower Bound	Upper Bound
1	2	-.056*	.013	.000	-.083	-.029
	3	-.087*	.014	.000	-.114	-.059
	4	-.096*	.013	.000	-.122	-.071
2	1	.056*	.013	.000	.029	.083
	3	-.030*	.009	.002	-.049	-.012
	4	-.040*	.009	.000	-.057	-.022
3	1	.087*	.014	.000	.059	.114
	2	.030*	.009	.002	.012	.049
	4	-.010	.007	.193	-.024	.005
4	1	.096*	.013	.000	.071	.122
	2	.040*	.009	.000	.022	.057
	3	.010	.007	.193	-.005	.024

Based on estimated marginal means

*. The mean difference is significant at the .05 level.

a. Adjustment for multiple comparisons: Least Significant Difference (equivalent to no adjustments).

Multivariate Tests

	Value	F	Hypothesis df	Error df	Sig.	Partial Eta Squared	Noncent. Parameter	Observed Power[b]
Pillai's trace	.658	21.128[a]	3.000	33.000	.000	.658	63.384	1.000
Wilks' lambda	.342	21.128[a]	3.000	33.000	.000	.658	63.384	1.000
Hotelling's trace	1.921	21.128[a]	3.000	33.000	.000	.658	63.384	1.000
Roy's largest root	1.921	21.128[a]	3.000	33.000	.000	.658	63.384	1.000

Each F tests the multivariate effect of Test. These tests are based on the linearly independent pairwise comparisons among the estimated marginal means.

a. Exact statistic

b. Computed using alpha = .05

3. Group * Test

Measure: MEASURE_1

Group	Test	Mean	Std. Error	95% Confidence Interval	
				Lower Bound	Upper Bound
.00	1	.573	.025	.521	.624
	2	.625	.018	.587	.662
	3	.664	.016	.631	.697
	4	.662	.017	.628	.695
1.00	1	.578	.026	.526	.631
	2	.639	.019	.601	.677
	3	.660	.017	.626	.694
	4	.682	.017	.647	.716

Profile Plots

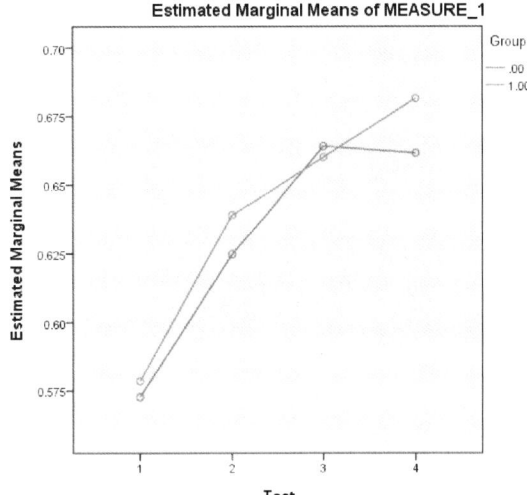

Appendix L

```
USE ALL.
COMPUTE filter_$=(Assessment=3 AND Train=1).
VARIABLE LABEL filter_$ 'Assessment=3 AND Train=1 (FILTER)'.
VALUE LABELS filter_$ 0 'Not Selected' 1 'Selected'.
FORMAT filter_$ (f1.0).
FILTER BY filter_$.
EXECUTE.
REGRESSION
  /DESCRIPTIVES MEAN STDDEV CORR SIG N
  /MISSING PAIRWISE
  /STATISTICS COEFF OUTS CI(95) R ANOVA COLLIN TOL CHANGE ZPP
  /CRITERIA=PIN(.05) POUT(.10)
  /NOORIGIN
  /DEPENDENT AI
  /METHOD=ENTER LogPP3_tot LogPP10_total
  /PARTIALPLOT ALL
  /SCATTERPLOT=(*ZRESID ,*ZPRED) (*SRESID ,*ZPRED)
  /RESIDUALS DURBIN HISTOGRAM(ZRESID) NORMPROB(ZRESID)
  /CASEWISE PLOT(ZRESID) OUTLIERS(3).
```

Regression

Notes

Output Created		15-Nov-2010 14:08:27
Comments		
Input	Data	F:\PASW_Sleep\SPSS\Means_final.sav
	Active Dataset	DataSet1
	Filter	Assessment=3 AND Train=1 (FILTER)
	Weight	<none>
	Split File	<none>
	N of Rows in Working Data File	40
Missing Value Handling	Definition of Missing	User-defined missing values are treated as missing.

	Cases Used	Correlation coefficients for each pair of variables are based on all the cases with valid data for that pair. Regression statistics are based on these correlations.

Syntax		REGRESSION
		  /DESCRIPTIVES MEAN STDDEV CORR SIG N
		  /MISSING PAIRWISE
		  /STATISTICS COEFF OUTS CI(95) R ANOVA COLLIN TOL CHANGE ZPP
		  /CRITERIA=PIN(.05) POUT(.10)
		  /NOORIGIN
		  /DEPENDENT AI
		  /METHOD=ENTER LogPP3_tot LogPP10_total
		  /PARTIALPLOT ALL
		  /SCATTERPLOT=(*ZRESID ,*ZPRED) (*SRESID ,*ZPRED)
		  /RESIDUALS DURBIN HISTOGRAM(ZRESID) NORMPROB(ZRESID)
		  /CASEWISE PLOT(ZRESID) OUTLIERS(3).

Resources	Processor Time	00:00:01.172
	Elapsed Time	00:00:01.219
	Memory Required	4748 bytes
	Additional Memory Required for Residual Plots	1880 bytes

[DataSet1] F:\PASW_Sleep\SPSS\Means_final.sav

Descriptive Statistics

	Mean	Std. Deviation	N
AI	.6088	.09678	40
LogPP3_tot	-.4939	.40426	39
LogPP10_total	.0348	.22728	39

Correlations

		AI	LogPP3_tot	LogPP10_total
Pearson Correlation	AI	1.000	-.347	-.383
	LogPP3_tot	-.347	1.000	.138
	LogPP10_total	-.383	.138	1.000
Sig. (1-tailed)	AI	.	.015	.008
	LogPP3_tot	.015	.	.201
	LogPP10_total	.008	.201	.
N	AI	40	39	39
	LogPP3_tot	39	39	39
	LogPP10_total	39	39	39

Variables Entered/Removed[b]

Model	Variables Entered	Variables Removed	Method
1	LogPP10_total, LogPP3_tot[a]	.	Enter

a. All requested variables entered.

b. Dependent Variable: AI

Model Summary[b]

Model	R	R Square	Adjusted R Square	Std. Error of the Estimate	Change Statistics					Durbin-Watson
					R Square Change	F Change	df1	df2	Sig. F Change	
1	.485[a]	.235	.192	.08698	.235	5.522	2	36	.008	2.191

a. Predictors: (Constant), LogPP10_total, LogPP3_tot

b. Dependent Variable: AI

ANOVA[b]

Model		Sum of Squares	df	Mean Square	F	Sig.
1	Regression	.084	2	.042	5.522	.008[a]
	Residual	.272	36	.008		
	Total	.356	38			

a. Predictors: (Constant), LogPP10_total, LogPP3_tot

b. Dependent Variable: AI

Coefficients[a]

Model		Unstandardized Coefficients		Standardized Coefficients	t	Sig.	95.0% Confidence Interval for B		Correlations			Collinearity Statistics	
		B	Std. Error	Beta			Lower Bound	Upper Bound	Zero-order	Partial	Part	Tolerance	VIF
1	(Constant)	.578	.023		25.556	.000	.532	.624					
	LogPP3_tot	-.072	.035	-.300	-2.039	.049	-.143	.000	-.347	-.322	-.297	.981	1.019
	LogPP10_total	-.145	.063	-.341	-2.318	.026	-.272	-.018	-.383	-.360	-.338	.981	1.019

Coefficients[a]

Model		Unstandardized Coefficients		Standardized Coefficients	t	Sig.	95.0% Confidence Interval for B		Correlations			Collinearity Statistics	
		B	Std. Error	Beta			Lower Bound	Upper Bound	Zero-order	Partial	Part	Tolerance	VIF
1	(Constant)	.578	.023		25.556	.000	.532	.624					
	LogPP3_tot	-.072	.035	-.300	-2.039	.049	-.143	.000	-.347	-.322	-.297	.981	1.019
	LogPP10_total	-.145	.063	-.341	-2.318	.026	-.272	-.018	-.383	-.360	-.338	.981	1.019

a. Dependent Variable: AI

Collinearity Diagnostics[a]

Model	Dimension	Eigenvalue	Condition Index	Variance Proportions		
				(Constant)	LogPP3_tot	LogPP10_total
1	1	1.800	1.000	.10	.10	.01
	2	.987	1.350	.00	.01	.93
	3	.213	2.907	.90	.88	.05

a. Dependent Variable: AI

Casewise Diagnostics[a]

Case Number	Std. Residual	AI	Predicted Value	Residual
7	-3.380	.31	.6003	-.29402
67	-3.391	.32	.6105	-.29499

a. Dependent Variable: AI

Residuals Statistics[a]

	Minimum	Maximum	Mean	Std. Deviation	N
Predicted Value	.5146	.7124	.6088	.04689	39
Std. Predicted Value	-2.009	2.210	.000	1.000	39
Standard Error of Predicted Value	.014	.045	.023	.007	39
Adjusted Predicted Value	.5030	.7190	.6081	.04729	39
Residual	-.29499	.13296	.00135	.08543	39
Std. Residual	-3.391	1.529	.016	.982	39
Stud. Residual	-3.477	1.624	.020	1.013	39
Deleted Residual	-.31095	.15005	.00210	.09094	39
Stud. Deleted Residual	-4.208	1.663	-.017	1.150	39
Mahal. Distance	.010	9.026	1.949	1.965	39
Cook's Distance	.000	.232	.022	.050	39
Centered Leverage Value	.000	.238	.051	.052	39

a. Dependent Variable: AI

Charts

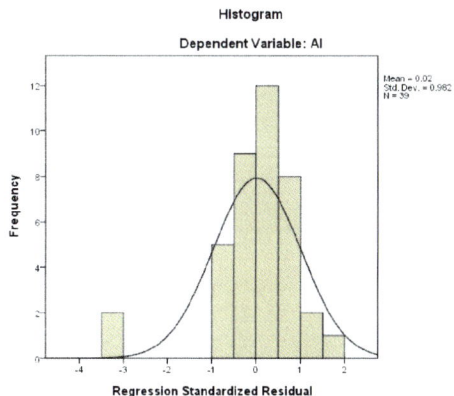

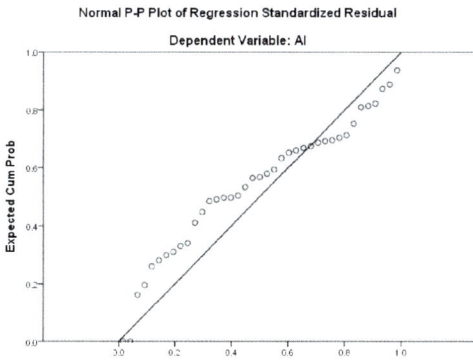

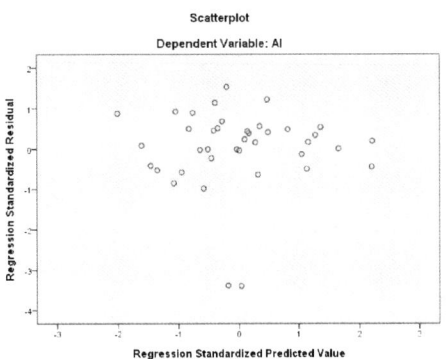

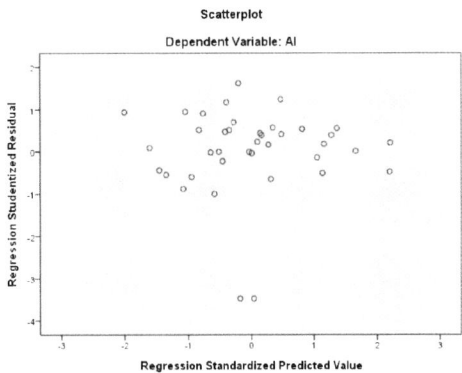

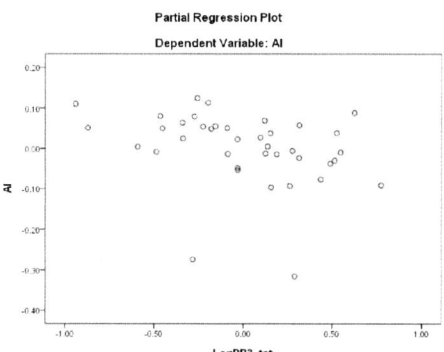

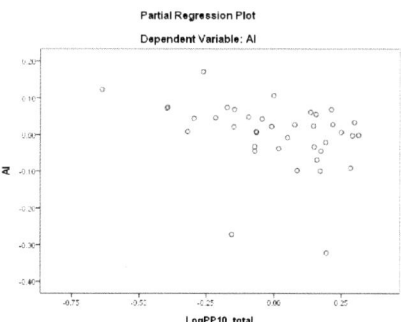

Regression: OR removed

Notes

Output Created		15-Nov-2010 14:09:58
Comments		
Input	Data	F:\PASW_Sleep\SPSS\Means_final.sav
	Active Dataset	DataSet1
	Filter	Assessment=3 AND Train=1 (FILTER)
	Weight	<none>
	Split File	<none>
	N of Rows in Working Data File	40
Missing Value Handling	Definition of Missing	User-defined missing values are treated as missing.
	Cases Used	Correlation coefficients for each pair of variables are based on all the cases with valid data for that pair. Regression statistics are based on these correlations.

Syntax		REGRESSION /DESCRIPTIVES MEAN STDDEV CORR SIG N /MISSING PAIRWISE /STATISTICS COEFF OUTS CI(95) R ANOVA COLLIN TOL CHANGE ZPP /CRITERIA=PIN(.05) POUT(.10) /NOORIGIN /DEPENDENT AI /METHOD=ENTER LogPP3_tot /METHOD=ENTER LogPP10_total /PARTIALPLOT ALL /SCATTERPLOT=(*ZRESID ,*ZPRED) (*SRESID ,*ZPRED) /RESIDUALS DURBIN HISTOGRAM(ZRESID) NORMPROB(ZRESID) /CASEWISE PLOT(ZRESID) OUTLIERS(3).
Resources	Processor Time	00:00:01.125
	Elapsed Time	00:00:01.140
	Memory Required	4804 bytes
	Additional Memory Required for Residual Plots	1880 bytes

[DataSet1] F:\PASW_Sleep\SPSS\Means_final.sav

Descriptive Statistics

Variables Entered/Removed[b]

Model	Variables Entered	Variables Removed	Method
1	LogPP3_tot[a]		Enter
2	LogPP10_total[a]		Enter

a. All requested variables entered.

b. Dependent Variable: AI

	Mean	Std. Deviation	N
AI	.6245	.06944	38
LogPP3_tot	-.4939	.40426	39
LogPP10_total	.0348	.22728	39

Correlations

		AI	LogPP3_tot	LogPP10_total
Pearson Correlation	AI	1.000	-.504	-.536
	LogPP3_tot	-.504	1.000	.138
	LogPP10_total	-.536	.138	1.000
Sig. (1-tailed)	AI	.	.001	.000
	LogPP3_tot	.001	.	.201
	LogPP10_total	.000	.201	.
N	AI	38	37	37
	LogPP3_tot	37	39	39
	LogPP10_total	37	39	39

Model Summary[c]

Model	R	R Square	Adjusted R	Std. Error of	Change Statistics					Durbin-
					R Square Change	F Change	df1	df2	Sig. F Change	

1	.504[a]	.254	.233	.06083	.254	11.913	1	35	.001	
2	.690[b]	.476	.445	.05172	.222	14.409	1	34	.001	2.273

a. Predictors: (Constant), LogPP3_tot

b. Predictors: (Constant), LogPP3_tot, LogPP10_total

c. Dependent Variable: AI

ANOVA[c]

Model		Sum of Squares	df	Mean Square	F	Sig.
1	Regression	.044	1	.044	11.913	.001[a]
	Residual	.130	35	.004		
	Total	.174	36			
2	Regression	.083	2	.041	15.443	.000[b]
	Residual	.091	34	.003		
	Total	.174	36			

a. Predictors: (Constant), LogPP3_tot

b. Predictors: (Constant), LogPP3_tot, LogPP10_total

c. Dependent Variable: AI

Coefficients[a]

Model		Unstandardized Coefficients		Standardized Coefficients	t	Sig.	95.0% Confidence Interval for B		Correlations			Collinearity Statistics	
		B	Std. Error	Beta			Lower Bound	Upper Bound	Zero-order	Partial	Part	Tolerance	VIF
	(Constant)	.582	.016		36.542	.000	.549	.614					

		B	Std. Error	Beta	t	Sig.	Zero-order	Partial	Part		Tolerance	VIF
	LogPP3_tot	-.087	.025	-.504	-3.452	.001	-.137	-.036	-.504	-.504	1.000	1.000
2	(Constant)	.592	.014		42.854	.000	.564	.620				
	LogPP3_tot	-.075	.022	-.438	-3.497	.001	-.119	-.032	-.504	-.514	.981	1.019
										-.434		
	LogPP10_total	-.145	.038	-.476	-3.796	.001	-.223	-.068	-.536	-.546	.981	1.019
										-.471		

a. Dependent Variable: AI

Excluded Variables[b]

Model						Collinearity Statistics		
		Beta In	t	Sig.	Partial Correlation	Tolerance	VIF	Minimum Tolerance
1	LogPP10_total	-.476[a]	-3.796	.001	-.546	.981	1.019	.981

a. Predictors in the Model: (Constant), LogPP3_tot

b. Dependent Variable: AI

Collinearity Diagnostics[a]

Model	Dimension	Eigenvalue	Condition Index	Variance Proportions		
				(Constant)	LogPP3_tot	LogPP10_total
1	1	1.778	1.000	.11	.11	
	2	.222	2.830	.89	.89	
2	1	1.800	1.000	.10	.10	.01
	2	.987	1.350	.00	.01	.93
	3	.213	2.909	.90	.88	.05

a. Dependent Variable: AI

Residuals Statistics[a]

	Minimum	Maximum	Mean	Std. Deviation	N
Predicted Value	.5282	.7301	.6245	.04791	39
Std. Predicted Value	-2.010	2.204	.000	1.000	39
Standard Error of Predicted Value	.009	.027	.014	.004	39
Adjusted Predicted Value	.5180	.7410	.6244	.05009	37
Residual	-.10058	.11922	.00167	.05080	37
Std. Residual	-1.944	2.305	.032	.982	37
Stud. Residual	-1.981	2.457	.035	1.022	37
Deleted Residual	-.10440	.13551	.00193	.05508	37
Stud. Deleted Residual	-2.075	2.670	.038	1.052	37
Mahal. Distance	.010	9.026	1.949	1.965	39
Cook's Distance	.000	.275	.029	.049	37
Centered Leverage Value	.000	.251	.054	.055	39

a. Dependent Variable: AI

Charts

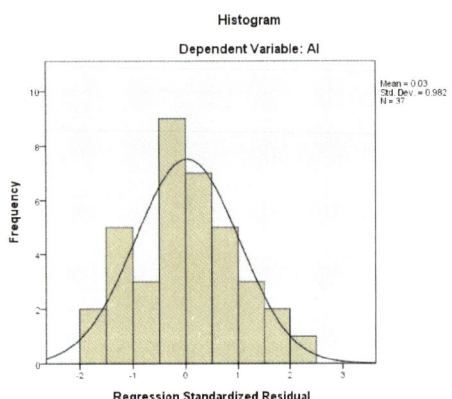

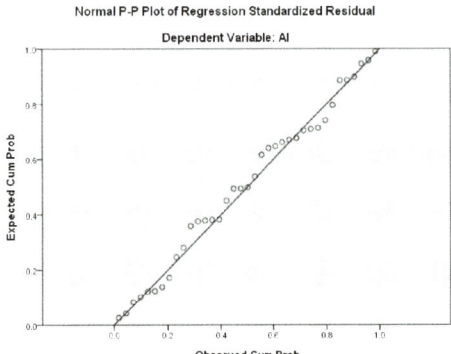

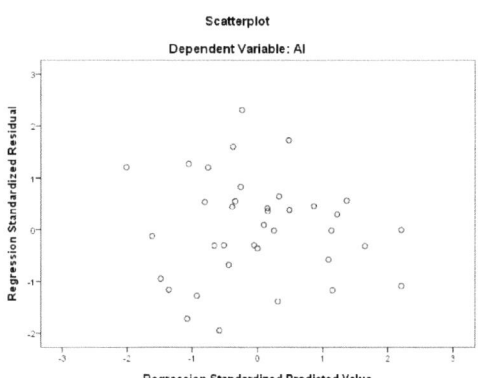

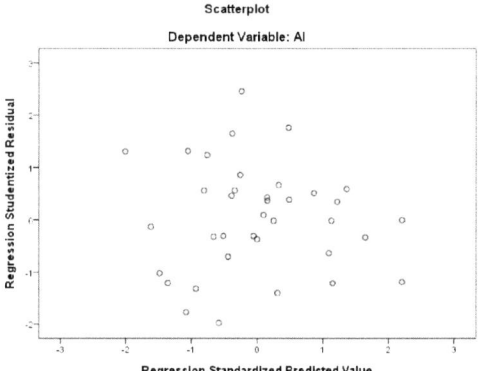

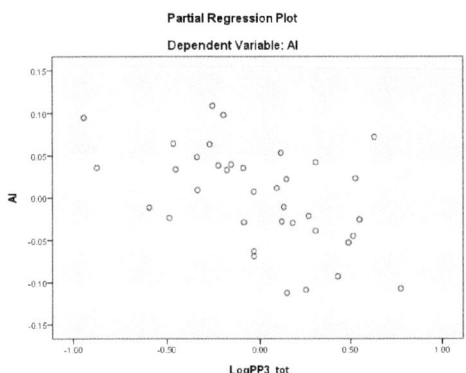

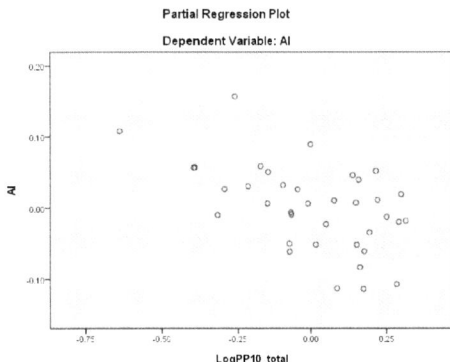

Appendix M

Day versus Night groups at baseline

Independent Samples Test

		Levene's Test for Equality of Variances		t-test for Equality of Means						
						Sig (2-tailed)	Mean Difference	Std. Error Difference	95% Confidence Interval of the Difference	
		F	Sig.	t	df				Lower	Upper
Age	Equal variances assumed	.000	.986	1.074	38	.290	1.300	1.211	-1.151	3.751
	Equal variances not assumed			1.074	37.944	.290	1.300	1.211	-1.151	3.751
LQ	Equal variances assumed	.011	.917	-.485	38	.630	-3.255	6.707	-16.833	10.323
	Equal variances not assumed			-.485	37.980	.630	-3.255	6.707	-16.833	10.323
PSQI_score_5_poor_sleeper	Equal variances assumed	2.365	.132	.931	38	.358	.600	.645	-.705	1.905
	Equal variances not assumed			.931	35.708	.358	.600	.645	-.708	1.908
ESS_score_10_sleepy_18_very_sleepy	Equal variances assumed	.646	.427	-1.012	38	.318	-1.150	1.136	-3.451	1.151
	Equal variances not assumed			-1.012	36.171	.318	-1.150	1.136	-3.454	1.154
SSS_pre	Equal variances assumed	.467	.499	-.760	38	.452	-.250	.329	-.916	.416
	Equal variances not assumed			-.760	36.856	.452	-.250	.329	-.917	.417
SSS_post	Equal variances assumed	.609	.440	-1.078	38	.288	-.400	.371	-1.151	.351
	Equal variances not assumed			-1.078	36.954	.288	-.400	.371	-1.152	.352
@_SSS_FU1	Equal variances assumed	.272	.605	-.772	37	.445	-.295	.382	-1.069	.479
	Equal variances not assumed			-.767	34.204	.448	-.295	.384	-1.076	.486
SSS_FU2	Equal variances assumed	.759	.389	1.393	37	.172	.371	.266	-.169	.911
	Equal variances not assumed			1.392	36.833	.172	.371	.266	-.169	.911

Skill versus movement groups at baseline

Independent Samples Test

		Levene's Test for Equality of Variances		t-test for Equality of Means						
						Sig (2-tailed)	Mean Difference	Std. Error Difference	95% Confidence Interval of the Difference	
		F	Sig.	t	df				Lower	Upper
Age	Equal variances assumed	10.590	.002	.992	48	.326	1.250	1.260	-1.283	3.783
	Equal variances not assumed			1.431	27.947	.164	1.250	.874	-.540	3.040
LQ	Equal variances assumed	.313	.578	1.563	48	.125	12.077	7.726	-3.457	27.612
	Equal variances not assumed			1.398	12.307	.187	12.077	8.637	-6.689	30.844
PSQI_score_5_poor_sleeper	Equal variances assumed	.022	.882	.480	48	.633	.350	.729	-1.115	1.815
	Equal variances not assumed			.462	13.242	.652	.350	.758	-1.285	1.985
ESS_score_10_sleepy_18_very_sleepy	Equal variances assumed	6.228	.016	.108	48	.915	.125	1.162	-2.211	2.461
	Equal variances not assumed			.180	42.269	.858	.125	.695	-1.277	1.527
SSS_pre	Equal variances assumed	.024	.878	-.627	48	.533	-.225	.359	-.946	.496
	Equal variances not assumed			-.675	15.259	.510	-.225	.334	-.935	.485
SSS_post	Equal variances assumed	.896	.349	-.124	48	.902	-.050	.403	-.860	.760
	Equal variances not assumed			-.140	16.379	.891	-.050	.358	-.807	.707
@_SSS_FU1	Equal variances assumed	4.789	.034	.372	47	.712	.144	.386	-.634	.921
	Equal variances not assumed			.573	34.747	.570	.144	.250	-.365	.652
SSS_FU2	Equal variances assumed	.068	.796	-.423	47	.675	-.131	.309	-.753	.492
	Equal variances not assumed			-.382	12.510	.709	-.131	.342	-.873	.611

Appendix N

Within-Subjects Factors

Measure:MEASURE_1

Test	Dependent Variable
1	AI_comp.1.00
2	AI_comp.2.00
3	AI_comp.3.00
4	AI_comp.4.00

Multivariate Tests[c]

Effect		Value	F	Hypothesis df	Error df	Sig.	Partial Eta Squared	Noncent. Parameter	Observed Power[b]
Test	Pillai's Trace	.658	21.128[a]	3.000	33.000	.000	.658	63.384	1.000
	Wilks' Lambda	.342	21.128[a]	3.000	33.000	.000	.658	63.384	1.000
	Hotelling's Trace	1.921	21.128[a]	3.000	33.000	.000	.658	63.384	1.000
	Roy's Largest Root	1.921	21.128[a]	3.000	33.000	.000	.658	63.384	1.000
Test * Group	Pillai's Trace	.079	.945[a]	3.000	33.000	.430	.079	2.836	.235
	Wilks' Lambda	.921	.945[a]	3.000	33.000	.430	.079	2.836	.235
	Hotelling's Trace	.086	.945[a]	3.000	33.000	.430	.079	2.836	.235
	Roy's Largest Root	.086	.945[a]	3.000	33.000	.430	.079	2.836	.235

a. Exact statistic

b. Computed using alpha = .05

c. Design: Intercept + Group

Within Subjects Design: Test

Mauchly's Test of Sphericity[b]

Measure:MEASURE_1

Within Subjects Effect	Mauchly's W	Approx. Chi-Square	df	Sig.	Epsilon[a]		
					Greenhouse-Geisser	Huynh-Feldt	Lower-bound
Test	.546	20.387	5	.001	.713	.783	.333

Tests the null hypothesis that the error covariance matrix of the orthonormalized transformed dependent variables is proportional to an identity matrix.

a. May be used to adjust the degrees of freedom for the averaged tests of significance. Corrected tests are displayed in the Tests of Within-Subjects Effects table.

b. Design: Intercept + Group

Within Subjects Design: Test

Tests of Within-Subjects Effects

Measure:MEASURE_1

Source		Type III Sum of Squares	df	Mean Square	F	Sig.	Partial Eta Squared	Noncent. Parameter	Observed Power[a]
Test	Sphericity Assumed	.208	3	.069	30.916	.000	.469	92.748	1.000
	Greenhouse-Geisser	.208	2.139	.097	30.916	.000	.469	66.140	1.000
	Huynh-Feldt	.208	2.348	.088	30.916	.000	.469	72.590	1.000
	Lower-bound	.208	1.000	.208	30.916	.000	.469	30.916	1.000
Test * Group	Sphericity Assumed	.003	3	.001	.448	.719	.013	1.343	.137
	Greenhouse-Geisser	.003	2.139	.001	.448	.654	.013	.958	.123
	Huynh-Feldt	.003	2.348	.001	.448	.672	.013	1.051	.126

	Lower-bound	.003	1.000	.003	.448	.508	.013	.448	.100
Error(Test)	Sphericity Assumed	.235	105	.002					
	Greenhouse-Geisser	.235	74.877	.003					
	Huynh-Feldt	.235	82.179	.003					
	Lower-bound	.235	35.000	.007					

a. Computed using alpha = .05

Estimates

Measure:MEASURE_1

Test	Mean	Std. Error	95% Confidence Interval	
			Lower Bound	Upper Bound
1	.576	.018	.539	.612
2	.632	.013	.605	.659
3	.662	.012	.638	.686
4	.672	.012	.647	.696

Pairwise Comparisons

Measure:MEASURE_1

(I) Test	(J) Test	Mean Difference (I-J)	Std. Error	Sig.^{a}	95% Confidence Interval for Difference^a	
					Lower Bound	Upper Bound
1	2	-.056*	.013	.000	-.083	-.029
	3	-.087*	.014	.000	-.114	-.059
	4	-.096*	.013	.000	-.122	-.071
2	1	.056*	.013	.000	.029	.083
	3	-.030*	.009	.002	-.049	-.012
	4	-.040*	.009	.000	-.057	-.022

3	1	.087*	.014	.000	.059	.114
	2	.030*	.009	.002	.012	.049
	4	-.010	.007	.193	-.024	.005
4	1	.096*	.013	.000	.071	.122
	2	.040*	.009	.000	.022	.057
	3	.010	.007	.193	-.005	.024

Based on estimated marginal means

*. The mean difference is significant at the .05 level.

a. Adjustment for multiple comparisons: Least Significant Difference (equivalent to no adjustments).

Appendix O

Within-Subjects Factors

Measure:MEASURE_1

Test	Dependent Variable
1	AI_incomp.1.00
2	AI_incomp.2.00
3	AI_incomp.3.00
4	AI_incomp.4.00

Multivariate Tests[c]

Effect		Value	F	Hypothesis df	Error df	Sig.	Partial Eta Squared	Noncent. Parameter	Observed Power[b]
Test	Pillai's Trace	.681	23.504[a]	3.000	33.000	.000	.681	70.511	1.000
	Wilks' Lambda	.319	23.504[a]	3.000	33.000	.000	.681	70.511	1.000

		Hotelling's Trace	2.137	23.504[a]	3.000	33.000	.000	.681	70.511	1.000
		Roy's Largest Root	2.137	23.504[a]	3.000	33.000	.000	.681	70.511	1.000
Test * Group	Pillai's Trace	.008	.092[a]	3.000	33.000	.964	.008	.275	.065
	Wilks' Lambda	.992	.092[a]	3.000	33.000	.964	.008	.275	.065
	Hotelling's Trace	.008	.092[a]	3.000	33.000	.964	.008	.275	.065
	Roy's Largest Root	.008	.092[a]	3.000	33.000	.964	.008	.275	.065

a. Exact statistic

b. Computed using alpha = .05

c. Design: Intercept + Group
Within Subjects Design: Test

Mauchly's Test of Sphericity[b]

Measure:MEASURE_1

Within Subjects Effect	Mauchly's W	Approx. Chi-Square	df	Sig.	Epsilon[a]		
					Greenhouse-Geisser	Huynh-Feldt	Lower-bound
Test	.685	12.767	5	.026	.808	.898	.333

Tests the null hypothesis that the error covariance matrix of the orthonormalized transformed dependent variables is proportional to an identity matrix.

a. May be used to adjust the degrees of freedom for the averaged tests of significance. Corrected tests are displayed in the Tests of Within-Subjects Effects table.

b. Design: Intercept + Group
Within Subjects Design: Test

Tests of Within-Subjects Effects

Measure:MEASURE_1

Source		Type III Sum of Squares	df	Mean Square	F	Sig.	Partial Eta Squared	Noncent. Parameter	Observed Power[a]
Test	Sphericity Assumed	.669	3	.223	28.206	.000	.446	84.618	1.000
	Greenhouse-Geisser	.669	2.425	.276	28.206	.000	.446	68.401	1.000
	Huynh-Feldt	.669	2.693	.248	28.206	.000	.446	75.961	1.000
	Lower-bound	.669	1.000	.669	28.206	.000	.446	28.206	.999
Test * Group	Sphericity Assumed	.003	3	.001	.117	.950	.003	.352	.071
	Greenhouse-Geisser	.003	2.425	.001	.117	.921	.003	.285	.069

	Huynh-Feldt	.003	2.693	.001	.117	.936	.003	.316	.070
	Lower-bound	.003	1.000	.003	.117	.734	.003	.117	.063
Error(Test)	Sphericity Assumed	.830	105	.008					
	Greenhouse-Geisser	.830	84.877	.010					
	Huynh-Feldt	.830	94.258	.009					
	Lower-bound	.830	35.000	.024					

a. Computed using alpha = .05

Estimates

Measure: MEASURE_1

Test	Mean	Std. Error	95% Confidence Interval	
			Lower Bound	Upper Bound
1	.427	.031	.364	.490
2	.508	.032	.444	.573
3	.574	.024	.526	.623
4	.602	.017	.567	.637

Pairwise Comparisons

Measure: MEASURE_1

(I) Test	(J) Test	Mean Difference (I-J)	Std. Error	Sig.[a]	95% Confidence Interval for Difference[a]	
					Lower Bound	Upper Bound
1	2	-.081*	.026	.003	-.133	-.029
	3	-.147*	.021	.000	-.190	-.104
	4	-.174*	.024	.000	-.222	-.127
2	1	.081*	.026	.003	.029	.133
	3	-.066*	.017	.000	-.100	-.031

		4	-.093*	.020	.000	-.133	-.054
3		1	.147*	.021	.000	.104	.190
		2	.066*	.017	.000	.031	.100
		4	-.028	.015	.078	-.058	.003
4		1	.174*	.024	.000	.127	.222
		2	.093*	.020	.000	.054	.133
		3	.028	.015	.078	-.003	.058

Based on estimated marginal means

*. The mean difference is significant at the .05 level.

a. Adjustment for multiple comparisons: Least Significant Difference (equivalent to no adjustments).

Appendix P

Within-Subjects Factors

Measure:MEASURE_1

Assessment	Dependent Variable
1	AI_comp.1.00
2	AI_comp.2.00
3	AI_comp.3.00
4	AI_comp.4.00

Multivariate Tests[c]

Effect		Value	F	Hypothesis df	Error df	Sig.	Partial Eta Squared	Noncent. Parameter	Observed Power[b]
Assessment	Pillai's Trace	.555	13.696[a]	3.000	33.000	.000	.555	41.088	1.000
	Wilks' Lambda	.445	13.696[a]	3.000	33.000	.000	.555	41.088	1.000
	Hotelling's Trace	1.245	13.696[a]	3.000	33.000	.000	.555	41.088	1.000
	Roy's Largest Root	1.245	13.696[a]	3.000	33.000	.000	.555	41.088	1.000
Assessment * Group	Pillai's Trace	.042	.476[a]	3.000	33.000	.701	.042	1.429	.136
	Wilks' Lambda	.958	.476[a]	3.000	33.000	.701	.042	1.429	.136
	Hotelling's Trace	.043	.476[a]	3.000	33.000	.701	.042	1.429	.136
	Roy's Largest Root	.043	.476[a]	3.000	33.000	.701	.042	1.429	.136

a. Exact statistic

b. Computed using alpha = .05

Multivariate Tests[c]

Effect		Value	F	Hypothesis df	Error df	Sig.	Partial Eta Squared	Noncent. Parameter	Observed Power[b]
Assessment	Pillai's Trace	.555	13.696[a]	3.000	33.000	.000	.555	41.088	1.000
	Wilks' Lambda	.445	13.696[a]	3.000	33.000	.000	.555	41.088	1.000
	Hotelling's Trace	1.245	13.696[a]	3.000	33.000	.000	.555	41.088	1.000
	Roy's Largest Root	1.245	13.696[a]	3.000	33.000	.000	.555	41.088	1.000
Assessment * Group	Pillai's Trace	.042	.476[a]	3.000	33.000	.701	.042	1.429	.136
	Wilks' Lambda	.958	.476[a]	3.000	33.000	.701	.042	1.429	.136
	Hotelling's Trace	.043	.476[a]	3.000	33.000	.701	.042	1.429	.136
	Roy's Largest Root	.043	.476[a]	3.000	33.000	.701	.042	1.429	.136

a. Exact statistic

b. Computed using alpha = .05

c. Design: Intercept + Group
Within Subjects Design: Assessment

Mauchly's Test of Sphericity

Measure:MEASURE_1

Within Subjects Effect	Mauchly's W	Approx. Chi-Square	df	Sig.	Epsilon[a]		
					Greenhouse-Geisser	Huynh-Feldt	Lower-bound

Multivariate Tests^c

Effect		Value	F	Hypothesis df	Error df	Sig.	Partial Eta Squared	Noncent. Parameter	Observed Power^b
Assessment	Pillai's Trace	.555	13.696^a	3.000	33.000	.000	.555	41.088	1.000
	Wilks' Lambda	.445	13.696^a	3.000	33.000	.000	.555	41.088	1.000
	Hotelling's Trace	1.245	13.696^a	3.000	33.000	.000	.555	41.088	1.000
	Roy's Largest Root	1.245	13.696^a	3.000	33.000	.000	.555	41.088	1.000
Assessment * Group	Pillai's Trace	.042	.476^a	3.000	33.000	.701	.042	1.429	.136
	Wilks' Lambda	.958	.476^a	3.000	33.000	.701	.042	1.429	.136
	Hotelling's Trace	.043	.476^a	3.000	33.000	.701	.042	1.429	.136
	Roy's Largest Root	.043	.476^a	3.000	33.000	.701	.042	1.429	.136

a. Exact statistic

b. Computed using alpha = .05

Assessment	.278	43.186	5	.000	.551	.591	.333

Tests the null hypothesis that the error covariance matrix of the orthonormalized transformed dependent variables is proportional to an identity matrix.

a. May be used to adjust the degrees of freedom for the averaged tests of significance. Corrected tests are displayed in the Tests of Within-Subjects Effects table.

Multivariate Tests[c]

Effect		Value	F	Hypothesis df	Error df	Sig.	Partial Eta Squared	Noncent. Parameter	Observed Power[b]
Assessment	Pillai's Trace	.555	13.696[a]	3.000	33.000	.000	.555	41.088	1.000
	Wilks' Lambda	.445	13.696[a]	3.000	33.000	.000	.555	41.088	1.000
	Hotelling's Trace	1.245	13.696[a]	3.000	33.000	.000	.555	41.088	1.000
	Roy's Largest Root	1.245	13.696[a]	3.000	33.000	.000	.555	41.088	1.000
Assessment * Group	Pillai's Trace	.042	.476[a]	3.000	33.000	.701	.042	1.429	.136
	Wilks' Lambda	.958	.476[a]	3.000	33.000	.701	.042	1.429	.136
	Hotelling's Trace	.043	.476[a]	3.000	33.000	.701	.042	1.429	.136
	Roy's Largest Root	.043	.476[a]	3.000	33.000	.701	.042	1.429	.136

a. Exact statistic

b. Computed using alpha = .05

b. Design: Intercept + Group
Within Subjects Design: Assessment

Tests of Within-Subjects Effects

Measure:MEASURE_1

Source		Type III Sum of Squares	df	Mean Square	F	Sig.	Partial Eta Squared	Noncent. Parameter	Observed Power[a]
Assessment	Sphericity Assumed	.984	3	.328	30.326	.000	.464	90.979	1.000
	Greenhouse-Geisser	.984	1.652	.596	30.326	.000	.464	50.106	1.000
	Huynh-Feldt	.984	1.773	.555	30.326	.000	.464	53.775	1.000
	Lower-bound	.984	1.000	.984	30.326	.000	.464	30.326	1.000
Assessment * Group	Sphericity Assumed	.023	3	.008	.697	.556	.020	2.092	.194
	Greenhouse-Geisser	.023	1.652	.014	.697	.476	.020	1.152	.152
	Huynh-Feldt	.023	1.773	.013	.697	.485	.020	1.236	.156
	Lower-bound	.023	1.000	.023	.697	.409	.020	.697	.128
Error(Assessment)	Sphericity Assumed	1.136	105	.011					
	Greenhouse-Geisser	1.136	57.828	.020					
	Huynh-Feldt	1.136	62.062	.018					
	Lower-bound	1.136	35.000	.032					

a. Computed using alpha = .05

Estimates

Measure:MEASURE_1

Assessment	Mean	Std. Error	95% Confidence Interval	
			Lower Bound	Upper Bound
1	.450	.035	.380	.520

2	.637	.014	.609	.666
3	.613	.017	.579	.648
4	.655	.011	.632	.677

Pairwise Comparisons

Measure:MEASURE_1

(I) Assessment	(J) Assessment	Mean Difference (I-J)	Std. Error	Sig.[a]	95% Confidence Interval for Difference[a]	
					Lower Bound	Upper Bound
1	2	-.188*	.033	.000	-.255	-.120
	3	-.164*	.027	.000	-.219	-.108
	4	-.205*	.031	.000	-.268	-.142
2	1	.188*	.033	.000	.120	.255
	3	.024	.016	.151	-.009	.057
	4	-.017	.016	.292	-.050	.015
3	1	.164*	.027	.000	.108	.219
	2	-.024	.016	.151	-.057	.009
	4	-.041*	.013	.003	-.068	-.015
4	1	.205*	.031	.000	.142	.268
	2	.017	.016	.292	-.015	.050
	3	.041*	.013	.003	.015	.068

Based on estimated marginal means

*. The mean difference is significant at the .05 level.

a. Adjustment for multiple comparisons: Least Significant Difference (equivalent to no adjustments).

Appendix Q

Within-Subjects Factors

Measure:MEASURE_1

Assessment	Dependent Variable
1	AI_incomp.1.00
2	AI_incomp.2.00
3	AI_incomp.3.00
4	AI_incomp.4.00

Multivariate Tests^c

Effect		Value	F	Hypothesis df	Error df	Sig.	Partial Eta Squared	Noncent. Parameter	Observed Power[b]
Assessment	Pillai's Trace	.682	23.596[a]	3.000	33.000	.000	.682	70.788	1.000
	Wilks' Lambda	.318	23.596[a]	3.000	33.000	.000	.682	70.788	1.000
	Hotelling's Trace	2.145	23.596[a]	3.000	33.000	.000	.682	70.788	1.000
	Roy's Largest Root	2.145	23.596[a]	3.000	33.000	.000	.682	70.788	1.000
Assessment * Group	Pillai's Trace	.103	1.263[a]	3.000	33.000	.303	.103	3.788	.306
	Wilks' Lambda	.897	1.263[a]	3.000	33.000	.303	.103	3.788	.306
	Hotelling's Trace	.115	1.263[a]	3.000	33.000	.303	.103	3.788	.306
	Roy's Largest Root	.115	1.263[a]	3.000	33.000	.303	.103	3.788	.306

a. Exact statistic

b. Computed using alpha = .05

Tests of Within-Subjects Effects

Measure:MEASURE_1

Source		Type III Sum of Squares	df	Mean Square	F	Sig.	Partial Eta Squared	Noncent. Parameter	Observed Power[a]
Assessment	Sphericity Assumed	5.085	3	1.695	51.678	.000	.596	155.034	1.000
	Greenhouse-Geisser	5.085	1.906	2.668	51.678	.000	.596	98.481	1.000
	Huynh-Feldt	5.085	2.070	2.456	51.678	.000	.596	106.981	1.000
	Lower-bound	5.085	1.000	5.085	51.678	.000	.596	51.678	1.000
Assessment * Group	Sphericity Assumed	.263	3	.088	2.677	.051	.071	8.031	.638
	Greenhouse-Geisser	.263	1.906	.138	2.677	.079	.071	5.102	.501
	Huynh-Feldt	.263	2.070	.127	2.677	.074	.071	5.542	.524
	Lower-bound	.263	1.000	.263	2.677	.111	.071	2.677	.356
Error(Assessment)	Sphericity Assumed	3.444	105	.033					
	Greenhouse-Geisser	3.444	66.698	.052					
	Huynh-Feldt	3.444	72.455	.048					
	Lower-bound	3.444	35.000	.098					

a. Computed using alpha = .05

c. Design: Intercept + Group
 Within Subjects Design: Assessment

Estimates

Measure:MEASURE_1

Assessment	Mean	Std. Error	95% Confidence Interval	
			Lower Bound	Upper Bound
1	.082	.061	-.042	.205
2	.476	.040	.395	.557
3	.500	.030	.438	.562
4	.543	.024	.494	.592

Pairwise Comparisons

Measure:MEASURE_1

(I) Assessment	(J) Assessment	Mean Difference (I-J)	Std. Error	Sig.[a]	95% Confidence Interval for Difference[a]	
					Lower Bound	Upper Bound
1	2	-.394*	.050	.000	-.496	-.292
	3	-.418*	.051	.000	-.523	-.314
	4	-.461*	.054	.000	-.572	-.351
2	1	.394*	.050	.000	.292	.496
	3	-.024	.030	.436	-.086	.038
	4	-.067*	.030	.031	-.128	-.007
3	1	.418*	.051	.000	.314	.523
	2	.024	.030	.436	-.038	.086
	4	-.043	.027	.116	-.097	.011
4	1	.461*	.054	.000	.351	.572
	2	.067*	.030	.031	.007	.128
	3	.043	.027	.116	-.011	.097

Based on estimated marginal means

*. The mean difference is significant at the .05 level.

Pairwise Comparisons

Measure:MEASURE_1

(I) Assessment	(J) Assessment	Mean Difference (I-J)	Std. Error	Sig.[a]	95% Confidence Interval for Difference[a]	
					Lower Bound	Upper Bound
1	2	-.394*	.050	.000	-.496	-.292
	3	-.418*	.051	.000	-.523	-.314
	4	-.461*	.054	.000	-.572	-.351
2	1	.394*	.050	.000	.292	.496
	3	-.024	.030	.436	-.086	.038
	4	-.067*	.030	.031	-.128	-.007
3	1	.418*	.051	.000	.314	.523
	2	.024	.030	.436	-.038	.086
	4	-.043	.027	.116	-.097	.011
4	1	.461*	.054	.000	.351	.572
	2	.067*	.030	.031	.007	.128
	3	.043	.027	.116	-.011	.097

Based on estimated marginal means

*. The mean difference is significant at the .05 level.

a. Adjustment for multiple comparisons: Least Significant Difference (equivalent to no adjustments).

3. Group * Assessment

Measure:MEASURE_1

Group	Assessment	Mean	Std. Error	95% Confidence Interval	
				Lower Bound	Upper Bound
.00	1	.182	.085	.010	.354

	2	.481	.055	.369	.594
	3	.501	.043	.415	.588
	4	.546	.034	.477	.614
1.00	1	-.019	.087	-.196	.158
	2	.470	.057	.355	.586
	3	.499	.044	.410	.587
	4	.541	.034	.471	.611

Appendix R

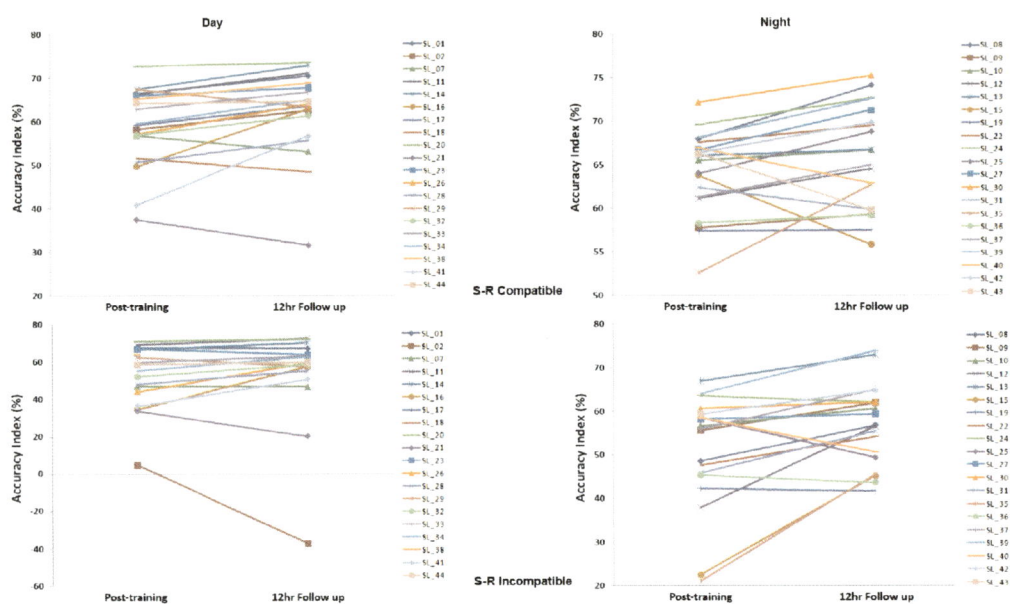

Appendix S

Within-Subjects Factors

Measure:MEASURE_1

Assessment	Dependent Variable
1	AI_incomp.1.00
2	AI_incomp.2.00
3	AI_incomp.3.00
4	AI_incomp.4.00

Multivariate Tests[c]

Effect		Value	F	Hypothesis df	Error df	Sig.	Partial Eta Squared	Noncent. Parameter	Observed Power[b]
Assessment	Pillai's Trace	.682	23.596[a]	3.000	33.000	.000	.682	70.788	1.000
	Wilks' Lambda	.318	23.596[a]	3.000	33.000	.000	.682	70.788	1.000
	Hotelling's Trace	2.145	23.596[a]	3.000	33.000	.000	.682	70.788	1.000
	Roy's Largest Root	2.145	23.596[a]	3.000	33.000	.000	.682	70.788	1.000
Assessment * Group	Pillai's Trace	.103	1.263[a]	3.000	33.000	.303	.103	3.788	.306
	Wilks' Lambda	.897	1.263[a]	3.000	33.000	.303	.103	3.788	.306
	Hotelling's Trace	.115	1.263[a]	3.000	33.000	.303	.103	3.788	.306
	Roy's Largest Root	.115	1.263[a]	3.000	33.000	.303	.103	3.788	.306

a. Exact statistic

b. Computed using alpha = .05

c. Design: Intercept + Group

Within Subjects Design: Assessment

Mauchly's Test of Sphericity[b]

Measure:MEASURE_1

Within Subjects Effect	Mauchly's W	Approx. Chi-Square	df	Sig.	Epsilon[a]		
					Greenhouse-Geisser	Huynh-Feldt	Lower-bound
Assessment	.437	27.891	5	.000	.635	.690	.333

Tests the null hypothesis that the error covariance matrix of the orthonormalized transformed dependent variables is proportional to an identity matrix.

a. May be used to adjust the degrees of freedom for the averaged tests of significance. Corrected tests are displayed in the Tests of Within-Subjects Effects table.

b. Design: Intercept + Group

Within Subjects Design: Assessment

Tests of Within-Subjects Effects

Measure:MEASURE_1

Source		Type III Sum of Squares	df	Mean Square	F	Sig.	Partial Eta Squared	Noncent. Parameter	Observed Power[a]
Assessment	Sphericity Assumed	5.085	3	1.695	51.678	.000	.596	155.034	1.000
	Greenhouse-Geisser	5.085	1.906	2.668	51.678	.000	.596	98.481	1.000
	Huynh-Feldt	5.085	2.070	2.456	51.678	.000	.596	106.981	1.000
	Lower-bound	5.085	1.000	5.085	51.678	.000	.596	51.678	1.000
Assessment *	Sphericity Assumed	.263	3	.088	2.677	.051	.071	8.031	.638

	Greenhouse-Geisser	.263	1.906	.138	2.677	.079	.071	5.102	.501
	Huynh-Feldt	.263	2.070	.127	2.677	.074	.071	5.542	.524
	Lower-bound	.263	1.000	.263	2.677	.111	.071	2.677	.356
Error(Assessment)	Sphericity Assumed	3.444	105	.033					
	Greenhouse-Geisser	3.444	66.698	.052					
	Huynh-Feldt	3.444	72.455	.048					
	Lower-bound	3.444	35.000	.098					

a. Computed using alpha = .05

Estimates

Measure:MEASURE_1

Assessment	Mean	Std. Error	95% Confidence Interval	
			Lower Bound	Upper Bound
1	.082	.061	-.042	.205
2	.476	.040	.395	.557
3	.500	.030	.438	.562
4	.543	.024	.494	.592

Pairwise Comparisons

Measure:MEASURE_1

(I) Assessment	(J) Assessment	Mean Difference (I-J)	Std. Error	Sig.[a]	95% Confidence Interval for Difference[a]	
					Lower Bound	Upper Bound
1	2	-.394*	.050	.000	-.535	-.254
	3	-.418*	.051	.000	-.562	-.275

			Mean Difference	Std. Error	Sig.	Lower Bound	Upper Bound
		4	-.461*	.054	.000	-.613	-.309
	2	1	.394*	.050	.000	.254	.535
		3	-.024	.030	1.000	-.109	.061
		4	-.067	.030	.184	-.151	.016
	3	1	.418*	.051	.000	.275	.562
		2	.024	.030	1.000	-.061	.109
		4	-.043	.027	.695	-.118	.032
	4	1	.461*	.054	.000	.309	.613
		2	.067	.030	.184	-.016	.151
		3	.043	.027	.695	-.032	.118

Based on estimated marginal means

*. The mean difference is significant at the .05 level.

a. Adjustment for multiple comparisons: Bonferroni.

3. Group * Assessment

Measure:MEASURE_1

Group	Assessment	Mean	Std. Error	95% Confidence Interval	
				Lower Bound	Upper Bound
.00	1	.182	.085	.010	.354
	2	.481	.055	.369	.594
	3	.501	.043	.415	.588
	4	.546	.034	.477	.614
1.00	1	-.019	.087	-.196	.158
	2	.470	.057	.355	.586
	3	.499	.044	.410	.587

Appendix T

Within-Subjects Factors

Measure:MEASURE_1

Assessment	Dependent Variable
1	Lag_incomp.1.00
2	Lag_incomp.2.00
3	Lag_incomp.3.00
4	Lag_incomp.4.00

Multivariate Tests[c]

Effect		Value	F	Hypothesis df	Error df	Sig.	Partial Eta Squared	Noncent. Parameter	Observed Power[b]
Assessment	Pillai's Trace	.235	3.371[a]	3.000	33.000	.030	.235	10.112	.710
	Wilks' Lambda	.765	3.371[a]	3.000	33.000	.030	.235	10.112	.710
	Hotelling's Trace	.306	3.371[a]	3.000	33.000	.030	.235	10.112	.710
	Roy's Largest Root	.306	3.371[a]	3.000	33.000	.030	.235	10.112	.710
Assessment * Group	Pillai's Trace	.062	.731[a]	3.000	33.000	.541	.062	2.193	.188
	Wilks' Lambda	.938	.731[a]	3.000	33.000	.541	.062	2.193	.188

	Hotelling's Trace	.066	.731[a]	3.000	33.000	.541	.062	2.193	.188
	Roy's Largest Root	.066	.731[a]	3.000	33.000	.541	.062	2.193	.188

a. Exact statistic

b. Computed using alpha = .05

c. Design: Intercept + Group
 Within Subjects Design: Assessment

Mauchly's Test of Sphericity[b]

Measure:MEASURE_1

Within Subjects Effect	Mauchly's W	Approx. Chi-Square	df	Sig.	Epsilon[a]		
					Greenhouse-Geisser	Huynh-Feldt	Lower-bound
Assessment	.339	36.445	5	.000	.602	.650	.333

Tests the null hypothesis that the error covariance matrix of the orthonormalized transformed dependent variables is proportional to an identity matrix.

a. May be used to adjust the degrees of freedom for the averaged tests of significance. Corrected tests are displayed in the Tests of Within-Subjects Effects table.

b. Design: Intercept + Group
 Within Subjects Design: Assessment

Tests of Within-Subjects Effects

Measure:MEASURE_1

Source		Type III Sum of Squares	df	Mean Square	F	Sig.	Partial Eta Squared	Noncent. Parameter	Observed Power[a]
Assessment	Sphericity Assumed	.740	3	.247	6.493	.000	.156	19.479	.966

	Greenhouse-Geisser	.740	1.805	.410	6.493	.004	.156	11.717	.870
	Huynh-Feldt	.740	1.951	.379	6.493	.003	.156	12.669	.889
	Lower-bound	.740	1.000	.740	6.493	.015	.156	6.493	.698
Assessment * Group	Sphericity Assumed	.172	3	.057	1.507	.217	.041	4.522	.388
	Greenhouse-Geisser	.172	1.805	.095	1.507	.230	.041	2.720	.295
	Huynh-Feldt	.172	1.951	.088	1.507	.229	.041	2.941	.307
	Lower-bound	.172	1.000	.172	1.507	.228	.041	1.507	.223
Error(Assessment)	Sphericity Assumed	3.988	105	.038					
	Greenhouse-Geisser	3.988	63.160	.063					
	Huynh-Feldt	3.988	68.290	.058					
	Lower-bound	3.988	35.000	.114					

a. Computed using alpha = .05

Estimates

Measure:MEASURE_1

Assessment	Mean	Std. Error	95% Confidence Interval	
			Lower Bound	Upper Bound
1	.232	.057	.116	.347
2	.120	.035	.049	.192
3	.064	.028	.006	.122
4	.054	.026	.002	.105

Pairwise Comparisons

Measure:MEASURE_1

(I) Assessment	(J) Assessment	Mean Difference (I-J)	Std. Error	Sig.[a]	95% Confidence Interval for Difference[a]	
					Lower Bound	Upper Bound
1	2	.111	.052	.240	-.035	.257
	3	.168*	.055	.026	.014	.321
	4	.178*	.061	.036	.008	.349
2	1	-.111	.052	.240	-.257	.035
	3	.057	.035	.694	-.042	.155
	4	.067	.028	.131	-.011	.145
3	1	-.168*	.055	.026	-.321	-.014
	2	-.057	.035	.694	-.155	.042
	4	.010	.030	1.000	-.072	.093
4	1	-.178*	.061	.036	-.349	-.008
	2	-.067	.028	.131	-.145	.011
	3	-.010	.030	1.000	-.093	.072

Based on estimated marginal means

a. Adjustment for multiple comparisons: Bonferroni.

*. The mean difference is significant at the .05 level.

Appendix U

Within-Subjects Factors

Measure:MEASURE_1

test	Dependent Variable
1	AI_Mean.2.00
2	AI_Mean.5.00

Multivariate Tests[c]

Effect		Value	F	Hypothesis df	Error df	Sig.	Partial Eta Squared	Noncent. Parameter	Observed Power[b]
test	Pillai's Trace	.814	161.826[a]	1.000	37.000	.000	.814	161.826	1.000
	Wilks' Lambda	.186	161.826[a]	1.000	37.000	.000	.814	161.826	1.000
	Hotelling's Trace	4.374	161.826[a]	1.000	37.000	.000	.814	161.826	1.000
	Roy's Largest Root	4.374	161.826[a]	1.000	37.000	.000	.814	161.826	1.000
test * Group	Pillai's Trace	.014	.525[a]	1.000	37.000	.473	.014	.525	.109
	Wilks' Lambda	.986	.525[a]	1.000	37.000	.473	.014	.525	.109
	Hotelling's Trace	.014	.525[a]	1.000	37.000	.473	.014	.525	.109
	Roy's Largest Root	.014	.525[a]	1.000	37.000	.473	.014	.525	.109

a. Exact statistic

b. Computed using alpha = .05

c. Design: Intercept + Group
Within Subjects Design: test

Tests of Within-Subjects Effects

Measure:MEASURE_1

Source		Type III Sum of Squares	df	Mean Square	F	Sig.	Partial Eta Squared	Noncent. Parameter	Observed Power[a]
test	Sphericity Assumed	.232	1	.232	161.826	.000	.814	161.826	1.000
	Greenhouse-Geisser	.232	1.000	.232	161.826	.000	.814	161.826	1.000
	Huynh-Feldt	.232	1.000	.232	161.826	.000	.814	161.826	1.000
	Lower-bound	.232	1.000	.232	161.826	.000	.814	161.826	1.000
test * Group	Sphericity Assumed	.001	1	.001	.525	.473	.014	.525	.109
	Greenhouse-Geisser	.001	1.000	.001	.525	.473	.014	.525	.109
	Huynh-Feldt	.001	1.000	.001	.525	.473	.014	.525	.109
	Lower-bound	.001	1.000	.001	.525	.473	.014	.525	.109
Error(test)	Sphericity Assumed	.053	37	.001					
	Greenhouse-Geisser	.053	37.000	.001					
	Huynh-Feldt	.053	37.000	.001					
	Lower-bound	.053	37.000	.001					

a. Computed using alpha = .05

Estimates

Measure:MEASURE_1

test	Mean	Std. Error	95% Confidence Interval	
			Lower Bound	Upper Bound
1	.434	.016	.401	.467
2	.543	.011	.521	.565

Pairwise Comparisons

Measure:MEASURE_1

(I) test	(J) test	Mean Difference (I-J)	Std. Error	Sig.[a]	95% Confidence Interval for Difference[a]	
					Lower Bound	Upper Bound
1	2	-.109[*]	.009	.000	-.126	-.092
2	1	.109[*]	.009	.000	.092	.126

Based on estimated marginal means

*. The mean difference is significant at the .05 level.

a. Adjustment for multiple comparisons: Bonferroni.

Within-Subjects Factors

Measure:MEASURE_1

TrainingBlock	Dependent Variable
1	Lag.2.00
2	Lag.5.00

Multivariate Tests[c]

Effect		Value	F	Hypothesis df	Error df	Sig.	Partial Eta Squared	Noncent. Parameter	Observed Power[b]
TrainingBlock	Pillai's Trace	.314	16.926[a]	1.000	37.000	.000	.314	16.926	.980
	Wilks' Lambda	.686	16.926[a]	1.000	37.000	.000	.314	16.926	.980
	Hotelling's Trace	.457	16.926[a]	1.000	37.000	.000	.314	16.926	.980
	Roy's Largest Root	.457	16.926[a]	1.000	37.000	.000	.314	16.926	.980
TrainingBlock * Group	Pillai's Trace	.006	.206[a]	1.000	37.000	.653	.006	.206	.073
	Wilks' Lambda	.994	.206[a]	1.000	37.000	.653	.006	.206	.073
	Hotelling's Trace	.006	.206[a]	1.000	37.000	.653	.006	.206	.073
	Roy's Largest Root	.006	.206[a]	1.000	37.000	.653	.006	.206	.073

a. Exact statistic

b. Computed using alpha = .05

c. Design: Intercept + Group
 Within Subjects Design: TrainingBlock

Tests of Within-Subjects Effects

Measure:MEASURE_1

Source		Type III Sum of Squares	df	Mean Square	F	Sig.	Partial Eta Squared	Noncent. Parameter	Observed Power[a]
TrainingBlock	Sphericity Assumed	.180	1	.180	16.926	.000	.314	16.926	.980
	Greenhouse-Geisser	.180	1.000	.180	16.926	.000	.314	16.926	.980
	Huynh-Feldt	.180	1.000	.180	16.926	.000	.314	16.926	.980
	Lower-bound	.180	1.000	.180	16.926	.000	.314	16.926	.980
TrainingBlock * Group	Sphericity Assumed	.002	1	.002	.206	.653	.006	.206	.073
	Greenhouse-Geisser	.002	1.000	.002	.206	.653	.006	.206	.073
	Huynh-Feldt	.002	1.000	.002	.206	.653	.006	.206	.073
	Lower-bound	.002	1.000	.002	.206	.653	.006	.206	.073
Error(TrainingBlock)	Sphericity Assumed	.394	37	.011					
	Greenhouse-Geisser	.394	37.000	.011					
	Huynh-Feldt	.394	37.000	.011					
	Lower-bound	.394	37.000	.011					

a. Computed using alpha = .05

Estimates

Measure:MEASURE_1

TrainingBlock	Mean	Std. Error	95% Confidence Interval	
			Lower Bound	Upper Bound
1	.171	.026	.118	.223

Estimates

Measure:MEASURE_1

TrainingBlock	Mean	Std. Error	95% Confidence Interval	
			Lower Bound	Upper Bound
1	.171	.026	.118	.223
2	.074	.013	.049	.100

Pairwise Comparisons

Measure:MEASURE_1

(I) TrainingBlock	(J) TrainingBlock	Mean Difference (I-J)	Std. Error	Sig.[a]	95% Confidence Interval for Difference[a]	
					Lower Bound	Upper Bound
1	2	.096*	.023	.000	.049	.144
2	1	-.096*	.023	.000	-.144	-.049

Based on estimated marginal means

*. The mean difference is significant at the .05 level.

a. Adjustment for multiple comparisons: Bonferroni.

Appendix V

Statistics

		MEP	MEP_log
N	Valid	4047	4047
	Missing	190	190
Mean		1.0364843	-.3853
Std. Error of Mean		.01433392	.01635
Median		.7508201	-.2866
Mode		.04280[a]	-3.15[a]
Std. Deviation		.91186724	1.04017
Variance		.832	1.082
Skewness		1.616	-.921
Std. Error of Skewness		.038	.038
Kurtosis		2.731	1.482
Std. Error of Kurtosis		.077	.077
Range		4.99405	6.75
Minimum		.00587	-5.14
Maximum		4.99992	1.61
Percentiles	2.5	.0463112	-3.0724
	97.5	3.6725872	1.3009

a. Multiple modes exist. The smallest value is shown

Statistics

		PP_ratio	PP_ratio_log
N	Valid	4060	4060
	Missing	180	180
Mean		.8231	-.3857
Std. Error of Mean		.01414	.00942
Median		.5355	-.2712
Mode		.02[a]	-1.75[a]
Std. Deviation		.90129	.60007
Variance		.812	.360
Skewness		2.242	-.679
Std. Error of Skewness		.038	.038
Kurtosis		7.996	-.153
Std. Error of Kurtosis		.077	.077
Range		8.99	3.30
Minimum		.00	-2.35
Maximum		9.00	.95
Percentiles	2.5	.0180	-1.7453
	97.5	3.2384	.5103

Appendix W

Between-Subjects Factors

		N
Group	0	1658
	1	1609
Session	1	827
	2	820
	3	820
	4	800
Pre_Post	1	1637
	2	1630

Tests of Between-Subjects Effects

Dependent Variable: MEP_log

Source	Type III Sum of Squares	df	Mean Square	F	Sig.
Corrected Model	40.434[a]	15	2.696	2.432	.002
Intercept	605.943	1	605.943	546.798	.000
Group	.310	1	.310	.279	.597
Session	3.933	3	1.311	1.183	.315
Pre_Post	3.773	1	3.773	3.405	.065
Group * Session	11.212	3	3.737	3.372	.018
Group * Pre_Post	13.679	1	13.679	12.344	.000
Session * Pre_Post	4.920	3	1.640	1.480	.218
Group * Session * Pre_Post	2.179	3	.726	.656	.579

Error	3602.649	3251	1.108	
Total	4250.101	3267		
Corrected Total	3643.082	3266		

a. R Squared = .011 (Adjusted R Squared = .007)

Estimates

Dependent Variable: MEP_log

Group	Session	Mean	Std. Error	95% Confidence Interval	
				Lower Bound	Upper Bound
0	1	-.325	.051	-.426	-.224
	2	-.545	.051	-.646	-.445
	3	-.463	.051	-.564	-.362
	4	-.351	.053	-.454	-.247
1	1	-.434	.052	-.536	-.332
	2	-.383	.053	-.487	-.280
	3	-.458	.053	-.561	-.355
	4	-.486	.053	-.589	-.383

Pairwise Comparisons

Dependent Variable: MEP_log

Group	(I) Session	(J) Session	Mean Difference (I-J)	Std. Error	Sig.ª	95% Confidence Interval for Differenceª	
						Lower Bound	Upper Bound
0	1	2	.220*	.073	.002	.077	.363
		3	.138	.073	.058	-.005	.280
		4	.025	.074	.732	-.119	.170
	2	1	-.220*	.073	.002	-.363	-.077
		3	-.082	.073	.257	-.225	.060
		4	-.195*	.074	.008	-.339	-.051
	3	1	-.138	.073	.058	-.280	.005
		2	.082	.073	.257	-.060	.225
		4	-.113	.074	.126	-.257	.032
	4	1	-.025	.074	.732	-.170	.119
		2	.195*	.074	.008	.051	.339
		3	.113	.074	.126	-.032	.257
1	1	2	-.051	.074	.493	-.196	.094
		3	.024	.074	.746	-.121	.169
		4	.052	.074	.484	-.093	.197
	2	1	.051	.074	.493	-.094	.196
		3	.075	.074	.316	-.071	.221
		4	.103	.074	.168	-.043	.249
	3	1	-.024	.074	.746	-.169	.121
		2	-.075	.074	.316	-.221	.071
		4	.028	.074	.708	-.118	.174
	4	1	-.052	.074	.484	-.197	.093
		2	-.103	.074	.168	-.249	.043
		3	-.028	.074	.708	-.174	.118

*. The mean difference is significant at the .050 level.

Estimates

Dependent Variable:MEP_log

Group	Pre_Post	Mean	Std. Error	95% Confidence Interval	
				Lower Bound	Upper Bound
0	1	-.520	.037	-.592	-.448
	2	-.322	.037	-.394	-.251
1	1	-.410	.037	-.482	-.337
	2	-.471	.037	-.544	-.398

Pairwise Comparisons

Dependent Variable:MEP_log

Group	(I) Pre_Post	(J) Pre_Post	Mean Difference (I-J)	Std. Error	Sig.[a]	95% Confidence Interval for Difference[a]	
						Lower Bound	Upper Bound
0	1	2	-.197*	.052	.000	-.299	-.096
	2	1	.197*	.052	.000	.096	.299
1	1	2	.061	.052	.242	-.041	.164

			-.061	.052	.242	-.164	.041
2	1						

Between-Subjects Factors

		N
Group	0	1658
	1	1609
Session	1	827
	2	820
	3	820
	4	800
Trial	1	161
	2	164
	3	164
	4	164
	5	164
	6	164
	7	164
	8	164
	9	164
	10	164
	11	163
	12	163
	13	163
	14	163
	15	163
	16	163

17	163
18	163
19	163
20	163

Tests of Between-Subjects Effects

Dependent Variable:MEP_log

Source	Type III Sum of Squares	df	Mean Square	F	Sig.
Corrected Model	189.094[a]	159	1.189	1.070	.265
Intercept	605.415	1	605.415	544.595	.000
Group	.309	1	.309	.278	.598
Session	3.991	3	1.330	1.197	.309
Trial	28.931	19	1.523	1.370	.131
Group * Session	11.208	3	3.736	3.361	.018
Group * Trial	34.866	19	1.835	1.651	.037
Session * Trial	62.071	57	1.089	.980	.519
Group * Session * Trial	46.803	57	.821	.739	.929
Error	3453.988	3107	1.112		
Total	4250.101	3267			
Corrected Total	3643.082	3266			

a. R Squared = .052 (Adjusted R Squared = .003)

Estimates

Dependent Variable:MEP_log

Group	Trial	Mean	Std. Error	95% Confidence Interval	
				Lower Bound	Upper Bound
0	1	-.252	.117	-.482	-.022

Tests of Between-Subjects Effects

Dependent Variable:MEP_log

Source	Type III Sum of Squares	df	Mean Square	F	Sig.
Corrected Model	189.094[a]	159	1.189	1.070	.265
Intercept	605.415	1	605.415	544.595	.000
Group	.309	1	.309	.278	.598
Session	3.991	3	1.330	1.197	.309
Trial	28.931	19	1.523	1.370	.131
Group * Session	11.208	3	3.736	3.361	.018
Group * Trial	34.866	19	1.835	1.651	.037
Session * Trial	62.071	57	1.089	.980	.519
Group * Session * Trial	46.803	57	.821	.739	.929
Error	3453.988	3107	1.112		
Total	4250.101	3267			
Corrected Total	3643.082	3266			
2	-.444	.116	-.671	-.217	
3	-.766	.116	-.993	-.539	
4	-.338	.116	-.565	-.111	
5	-.360	.116	-.587	-.133	
6	-.568	.116	-.795	-.341	
7	-.501	.116	-.728	-.274	
8	-.645	.116	-.872	-.418	
9	-.679	.116	-.906	-.452	
10	-.641	.116	-.868	-.414	
11	-.390	.116	-.617	-.163	
12	-.352	.116	-.579	-.125	

Tests of Between-Subjects Effects

Dependent Variable:MEP_log

Source	Type III Sum of Squares	df	Mean Square	F	Sig.
Corrected Model	189.094[a]	159	1.189	1.070	.265
Intercept	605.415	1	605.415	544.595	.000
Group	.309	1	.309	.278	.598
Session	3.991	3	1.330	1.197	.309
Trial	28.931	19	1.523	1.370	.131
Group * Session	11.208	3	3.736	3.361	.018
Group * Trial	34.866	19	1.835	1.651	.037
Session * Trial	62.071	57	1.089	.980	.519
Group * Session * Trial	46.803	57	.821	.739	.929
Error	3453.988	3107	1.112		
Total	4250.101	3267			
Corrected Total	3643.082	3266			
	13	-.249	.116	-.476	-.022
	14	-.402	.116	-.629	-.175
	15	-.388	.116	-.615	-.161
	16	-.270	.116	-.497	-.043
	17	-.329	.116	-.555	-.102
	18	-.296	.116	-.523	-.069
	19	-.247	.116	-.474	-.020
	20	-.301	.116	-.528	-.074
1	1	-.311	.118	-.542	-.080
	2	-.360	.117	-.590	-.130
	3	-.463	.117	-.693	-.233

Tests of Between-Subjects Effects

Dependent Variable:MEP_log

Source	Type III Sum of Squares	df	Mean Square	F	Sig.
Corrected Model	189.094[a]	159	1.189	1.070	.265
Intercept	605.415	1	605.415	544.595	.000
Group	.309	1	.309	.278	.598
Session	3.991	3	1.330	1.197	.309
Trial	28.931	19	1.523	1.370	.131
Group * Session	11.208	3	3.736	3.361	.018
Group * Trial	34.866	19	1.835	1.651	.037
Session * Trial	62.071	57	1.089	.980	.519
Group * Session * Trial	46.803	57	.821	.739	.929
Error	3453.988	3107	1.112		
Total	4250.101	3267			
Corrected Total	3643.082	3266			
4	-.347	.117	-.577	-.117	
5	-.395	.117	-.625	-.165	
6	-.526	.117	-.755	-.296	
7	-.429	.117	-.659	-.199	
8	-.501	.117	-.731	-.271	
9	-.375	.117	-.605	-.145	
10	-.388	.117	-.618	-.158	
11	-.172	.118	-.403	.059	
12	-.517	.118	-.748	-.286	
13	-.472	.118	-.703	-.241	
14	-.527	.118	-.758	-.296	

Tests of Between-Subjects Effects

Dependent Variable:MEP_log

Source	Type III Sum of Squares	df	Mean Square	F	Sig.
Corrected Model	189.094[a]	159	1.189	1.070	.265
Intercept	605.415	1	605.415	544.595	.000
Group	.309	1	.309	.278	.598
Session	3.991	3	1.330	1.197	.309
Trial	28.931	19	1.523	1.370	.131
Group * Session	11.208	3	3.736	3.361	.018
Group * Trial	34.866	19	1.835	1.651	.037
Session * Trial	62.071	57	1.089	.980	.519
Group * Session * Trial	46.803	57	.821	.739	.929
Error	3453.988	3107	1.112		
Total	4250.101	3267			
Corrected Total	3643.082	3266			
15	-.253	.118	-.485	-.022	
16	-.554	.118	-.785	-.323	
17	-.507	.118	-.738	-.276	
18	-.440	.118	-.671	-.209	
19	-.506	.118	-.737	-.275	
20	-.765	.118	-.996	-.534	

Appendix X

General Linear Model

Notes

Output Created		23-Nov-2010 14:22:49
Comments		
Input	Data	E:\PASW_Sleep\SPSS\SPSS Data Sheets\PP_full.sav
	Active Dataset	DataSet2
	Filter	Train=1 (FILTER)
	Weight	<none>
	Split File	<none>
	N of Rows in Working Data File	3440
Missing Value Handling	Definition of Missing	User-defined missing values are treated as missing.
	Cases Used	Statistics are based on all cases with valid data for all variables in the model.
Syntax		glm PP_total_log by Group Session Trial ISI /EMMEANS = tables(Group*ISI)compare(Group) /EMMEANS = tables(Trial) /EMMEANS = tables(Group).
Resources	Processor Time	00:00:01.844
	Elapsed Time	00:00:01.953

[DataSet2] E:\PASW_Sleep\SPSS\SPSS Data Sheets\PP_full.sav

Between-Subjects Factors

		N
Group	0	1660
	1	1620
Session	1	840
	2	820
	3	820
	4	800
Trial	1	328
	2	328

	3	328
	4	328
	5	328
	6	328
	7	328
	8	328
	9	328
	10	328
ISI	3	1640
	10	1640

Tests of Between-Subjects Effects

Dependent Variable: PP_total_log

Source	Type III Sum of Squares	df	Mean Square	F	Sig.
Corrected Model	308.525[a]	159	1.940	6.638	.000
Intercept	526.041	1	526.041	1799.484	.000
Group	4.605	1	4.605	15.753	.000
Session	.755	3	.252	.861	.461
Trial	5.852	9	.650	2.224	.018
ISI	252.666	1	252.666	864.323	.000
Group * Session	1.914	3	.638	2.182	.088
Group * Trial	1.467	9	.163	.558	.832
Group * ISI	17.135	1	17.135	58.617	.000
Session * Trial	4.847	27	.180	.614	.940
Session * ISI	.376	3	.125	.428	.733
Trial * ISI	1.326	9	.147	.504	.873
Group * Session * Trial	3.665	27	.136	.464	.992
Group * Session * ISI	.434	3	.145	.495	.686
Group * Trial * ISI	1.452	9	.161	.552	.837
Session * Trial * ISI	4.210	27	.156	.533	.977
Group * Session * Trial * ISI	6.334	27	.235	.803	.753
Error	912.066	3120	.292		
Total	1748.164	3280			
Corrected Total	1220.591	3279			

a. R Squared = .253 (Adjusted R Squared = .215)

Estimated Marginal Means

1. Group * ISI

Estimates

Dependent Variable:PP_total_log

Group	ISI	Mean	Std. Error	95% Confidence Interval	
				Lower Bound	Upper Bound
0	3	-.788	.019	-.825	-.751
	10	-.088	.019	-.125	-.051
1	3	-.568	.019	-.606	-.531
	10	-.158	.019	-.195	-.121

Pairwise Comparisons

Dependent Variable:PP_total_log

ISI	(I) Group	(J) Group	Mean Difference (I-J)	Std. Error	Sig.^{a}	95% Confidence Interval for Difference^a	
						Lower Bound	Upper Bound
3	0	1	-.220*	.027	.000	-.272	-.167
	1	0	.220*	.027	.000	.167	.272
10	0	1	.070*	.027	.009	.017	.122
	1	0	-.070*	.027	.009	-.122	-.017

Based on estimated marginal means

*. The mean difference is significant at the .050 level.

a. Adjustment for multiple comparisons: Least Significant Difference (equivalent to no adjustments).

Univariate Tests

Dependent Variable:PP_total_log

ISI		Sum of Squares	df	Mean Square	F	Sig.
3	Contrast	19.753	1	19.753	67.572	.000
	Error	912.066	3120	.292		
10	Contrast	1.987	1	1.987	6.797	.009
	Error	912.066	3120	.292		

Each F tests the simple effects of Group within each level combination of the other effects shown. These tests are based on the linearly independent pairwise comparisons among the estimated marginal means.

2. Trial

Dependent Variable:PP_total_log

Trial	Mean	Std. Error	95% Confidence Interval	
			Lower Bound	Upper Bound
1	-.462	.030	-.521	-.404
2	-.426	.030	-.485	-.368
3	-.430	.030	-.489	-.372
4	-.456	.030	-.514	-.397
5	-.382	.030	-.440	-.323
6	-.394	.030	-.453	-.336
7	-.370	.030	-.429	-.312
8	-.390	.030	-.449	-.331
9	-.313	.030	-.371	-.254
10	-.382	.030	-.441	-.323

3. Group

Dependent Variable:PP_total_log

Group	Mean	Std. Error	95% Confidence Interval	
			Lower Bound	Upper Bound
0	-.438	.013	-.464	-.412
1	-.363	.013	-.389	-.337

Appendix Y

Within-Subjects Factors

Measure:MEASURE_1

Assessment	Dependent Variable
1	PP3_total_log.1.00
2	PP3_total_log.2.00
3	PP3_total_log.3.00
4	PP3_total_log.4.00

Multivariate Tests[c]

Effect		Value	F	Hypothesis df	Error df	Sig.	Partial Eta Squared	Noncent. Parameter	Observed Power[b]
Assessment	Pillai's Trace	.049	.581[a]	3.000	34.000	.632	.049	1.742	.157
	Wilks' Lambda	.951	.581[a]	3.000	34.000	.632	.049	1.742	.157
	Hotelling's Trace	.051	.581[a]	3.000	34.000	.632	.049	1.742	.157
	Roy's Largest Root	.051	.581[a]	3.000	34.000	.632	.049	1.742	.157
Assessment * Group	Pillai's Trace	.061	.734[a]	3.000	34.000	.539	.061	2.201	.190
	Wilks' Lambda	.939	.734[a]	3.000	34.000	.539	.061	2.201	.190

	Hotelling's Trace	.065	.734[a]	3.000	34.000	.539	.061	2.201	.190
	Roy's Largest Root	.065	.734[a]	3.000	34.000	.539	.061	2.201	.190

a. Exact statistic

b. Computed using alpha = .05

c. Design: Intercept + Group
   Within Subjects Design: Assessment

Tests of Within-Subjects Effects

Measure: MEASURE_1

Source		Type III Sum of Squares	df	Mean Square	F	Sig.	Partial Eta Squared	Noncent. Parameter	Observed Power[a]
Assessment	Sphericity Assumed	.109	3	.036	.600	.616	.016	1.800	.171
	Greenhouse-Geisser	.109	2.776	.039	.600	.604	.016	1.666	.166
	Huynh-Feldt	.109	3.000	.036	.600	.616	.016	1.800	.171
	Lower-bound	.109	1.000	.109	.600	.444	.016	.600	.117
Assessment * Group	Sphericity Assumed	.143	3	.048	.787	.504	.021	2.360	.215
	Greenhouse-Geisser	.143	2.776	.052	.787	.495	.021	2.184	.207
	Huynh-Feldt	.143	3.000	.048	.787	.504	.021	2.360	.215
	Lower-bound	.143	1.000	.143	.787	.381	.021	.787	.139
Error(Assessment)	Sphericity Assumed	6.565	108	.061					
	Greenhouse-Geisser	6.565	99.926	.066					
	Huynh-Feldt	6.565	108.000	.061					

	Lower-bound	6.565	36.000	.182				

a. Computed using alpha = .05

Tests of Between-Subjects Effects

Measure:MEASURE_1

Transformed Variable:Average

Source	Type III Sum of Squares	df	Mean Square	F	Sig.	Partial Eta Squared	Noncent. Parameter	Observed Power[a]
Intercept	33.769	1	33.769	100.638	.000	.737	100.638	1.000
Group	1.296	1	1.296	3.861	.057	.097	3.861	.481
Error	12.080	36	.336					

a. Computed using alpha = .05

1. Group

Measure:MEASURE_1

Group	Mean	Std. Error	95% Confidence Interval	
			Lower Bound	Upper Bound
0	-.564	.068	-.703	-.426
1	-.380	.065	-.511	-.248

Appendix Z

Within-Subjects Factors

Measure:MEASURE_1

test	Dependent Variable
1	rMT.1.00
2	rMT.2.00
3	rMT.3.00
4	rMT.4.00

Multivariate Tests[c]

Effect		Value	F	Hypothesis df	Error df	Sig.	Partial Eta Squared	Noncent. Parameter	Observed Power[b]
test	Pillai's Trace	.208	2.896[a]	3.000	33.000	.050	.208	8.688	.637
	Wilks' Lambda	.792	2.896[a]	3.000	33.000	.050	.208	8.688	.637
	Hotelling's Trace	.263	2.896[a]	3.000	33.000	.050	.208	8.688	.637
	Roy's Largest Root	.263	2.896[a]	3.000	33.000	.050	.208	8.688	.637
test * Group	Pillai's Trace	.219	3.085[a]	3.000	33.000	.041	.219	9.255	.667
	Wilks' Lambda	.781	3.085[a]	3.000	33.000	.041	.219	9.255	.667
	Hotelling's Trace	.280	3.085[a]	3.000	33.000	.041	.219	9.255	.667
	Roy's Largest Root	.280	3.085[a]	3.000	33.000	.041	.219	9.255	.667

a. Exact statistic

b. Computed using alpha = .05

Multivariate Tests[c]

Effect		Value	F	Hypothesis df	Error df	Sig.	Partial Eta Squared	Noncent. Parameter	Observed Power[b]
test	Pillai's Trace	.208	2.896[a]	3.000	33.000	.050	.208	8.688	.637
	Wilks' Lambda	.792	2.896[a]	3.000	33.000	.050	.208	8.688	.637
	Hotelling's Trace	.263	2.896[a]	3.000	33.000	.050	.208	8.688	.637
	Roy's Largest Root	.263	2.896[a]	3.000	33.000	.050	.208	8.688	.637
test * Group	Pillai's Trace	.219	3.085[a]	3.000	33.000	.041	.219	9.255	.667
	Wilks' Lambda	.781	3.085[a]	3.000	33.000	.041	.219	9.255	.667
	Hotelling's Trace	.280	3.085[a]	3.000	33.000	.041	.219	9.255	.667
	Roy's Largest Root	.280	3.085[a]	3.000	33.000	.041	.219	9.255	.667

a. Exact statistic

b. Computed using alpha = .05

c. Design: Intercept + Group
   Within Subjects Design: test

Mauchly's Test of Sphericity[b]

Measure:MEASURE_1

Within Subjects Effect	Mauchly's W	Approx. Chi-Square	df	Sig.	Epsilon[a]		
					Greenhouse-Geisser	Huynh-Feldt	Lower-bound
test	.583	18.194	5	.003	.774	.856	.333

Tests the null hypothesis that the error covariance matrix of the orthonormalized transformed dependent variables is proportional to an identity matrix.

a. May be used to adjust the degrees of freedom for the averaged tests of significance. Corrected tests are displayed in the Tests of Within-Subjects Effects table.

b. Design: Intercept + Group
Within Subjects Design: test

Tests of Within-Subjects Effects

Measure:MEASURE_1

Source		Type III Sum of Squares	df	Mean Square	F	Sig.	Partial Eta Squared	Noncent. Parameter	Observed Power[a]
test	Sphericity Assumed	84.658	3	28.219	4.955	.003	.124	14.865	.903
	Greenhouse-Geisser	84.658	2.322	36.457	4.955	.007	.124	11.506	.838
	Huynh-Feldt	84.658	2.568	32.966	4.955	.005	.124	12.725	.865
	Lower-bound	84.658	1.000	84.658	4.955	.033	.124	4.955	.581
test * Group	Sphericity Assumed	48.820	3	16.273	2.857	.041	.075	8.572	.670
	Greenhouse-Geisser	48.820	2.322	21.024	2.857	.055	.075	6.635	.588
	Huynh-Feldt	48.820	2.568	19.011	2.857	.049	.075	7.338	.619
	Lower-bound	48.820	1.000	48.820	2.857	.100	.075	2.857	.376
Error(test)	Sphericity Assumed	597.977	105	5.695					
	Greenhouse-Geisser	597.977	81.274	7.358					
	Huynh-Feldt	597.977	89.882	6.653					
	Lower-bound	597.977	35.000	17.085					

a. Computed using alpha = .05

Appendix AA

Within-Subjects Factors

Measure:MEASURE_1

test	Dependent Variable
1	aMT.1.00
2	aMT.2.00
3	aMT.3.00
4	aMT.4.00

Multivariate Tests[c]

Effect		Value	F	Hypothesis df	Error df	Sig.	Partial Eta Squared	Noncent. Parameter	Observed Power[b]
test	Pillai's Trace	.083	1.001[a]	3.000	33.000	.404	.083	3.004	.247
	Wilks' Lambda	.917	1.001[a]	3.000	33.000	.404	.083	3.004	.247
	Hotelling's Trace	.091	1.001[a]	3.000	33.000	.404	.083	3.004	.247
	Roy's Largest Root	.091	1.001[a]	3.000	33.000	.404	.083	3.004	.247
test * Group	Pillai's Trace	.030	.335[a]	3.000	33.000	.800	.030	1.004	.108
	Wilks' Lambda	.970	.335[a]	3.000	33.000	.800	.030	1.004	.108
	Hotelling's Trace	.030	.335[a]	3.000	33.000	.800	.030	1.004	.108
	Roy's Largest Root	.030	.335[a]	3.000	33.000	.800	.030	1.004	.108

a. Exact statistic

b. Computed using alpha = .05

Multivariate Tests^c

Effect		Value	F	Hypothesis df	Error df	Sig.	Partial Eta Squared	Noncent. Parameter	Observed Power[b]
test	Pillai's Trace	.083	1.001[a]	3.000	33.000	.404	.083	3.004	.247
	Wilks' Lambda	.917	1.001[a]	3.000	33.000	.404	.083	3.004	.247
	Hotelling's Trace	.091	1.001[a]	3.000	33.000	.404	.083	3.004	.247
	Roy's Largest Root	.091	1.001[a]	3.000	33.000	.404	.083	3.004	.247
test * Group	Pillai's Trace	.030	.335[a]	3.000	33.000	.800	.030	1.004	.108
	Wilks' Lambda	.970	.335[a]	3.000	33.000	.800	.030	1.004	.108
	Hotelling's Trace	.030	.335[a]	3.000	33.000	.800	.030	1.004	.108
	Roy's Largest Root	.030	.335[a]	3.000	33.000	.800	.030	1.004	.108

a. Exact statistic

b. Computed using alpha = .05

c. Design: Intercept + Group

Within Subjects Design: test

Mauchly's Test of Sphericity^b

Measure:MEASURE_1

Within Subjects Effect	Mauchly's W	Approx. Chi-Square	df	Sig.	Epsilon[a]		
					Greenhouse-Geisser	Huynh-Feldt	Lower-bound
test	.140	66.410	5	.000	.509	.543	.333

Tests the null hypothesis that the error covariance matrix of the orthonormalized transformed dependent variables is proportional to an identity matrix.

a. May be used to adjust the degrees of freedom for the averaged tests of significance. Corrected tests are displayed in the Tests of Within-Subjects Effects table.

Mauchly's Test of Sphericity[b]

Measure: MEASURE_1

Within Subjects Effect	Mauchly's W	Approx. Chi-Square	df	Sig.	Epsilon[a]		
					Greenhouse-Geisser	Huynh-Feldt	Lower-bound
test	.140	66.410	5	.000	.509	.543	.333

Tests the null hypothesis that the error covariance matrix of the orthonormalized transformed dependent variables is proportional to an identity matrix.

a. May be used to adjust the degrees of freedom for the averaged tests of significance. Corrected tests are displayed in the Tests of Within-Subjects Effects table.

b. Design: Intercept + Group
Within Subjects Design: test

Tests of Within-Subjects Effects

Measure: MEASURE_1

Source		Type III Sum of Squares	df	Mean Square	F	Sig.	Partial Eta Squared	Noncent. Parameter	Observed Power[a]
test	Sphericity Assumed	11.054	3	3.685	.405	.750	.011	1.214	.128
	Greenhouse-Geisser	11.054	1.527	7.238	.405	.614	.011	.618	.105
	Huynh-Feldt	11.054	1.628	6.788	.405	.627	.011	.659	.107
	Lower-bound	11.054	1.000	11.054	.405	.529	.011	.405	.095
test * Group	Sphericity Assumed	17.648	3	5.883	.646	.587	.018	1.939	.182
	Greenhouse-Geisser	17.648	1.527	11.556	.646	.488	.018	.987	.140
	Huynh-Feldt	17.648	1.628	10.838	.646	.497	.018	1.052	.143
	Lower-bound	17.648	1.000	17.648	.646	.427	.018	.646	.122
Error(test)	Sphericity Assumed	955.906	105	9.104					

	Greenhouse-Geisser	955.906	53.450	17.884
	Huynh-Feldt	955.906	56.991	16.773
	Lower-bound	955.906	35.000	27.312

a. Computed using alpha = .05

Tests of Between-Subjects Effects

Measure:MEASURE_1

Transformed Variable:Average

Source	Type III Sum of Squares	df	Mean Square	F	Sig.	Partial Eta Squared	Noncent. Parameter	Observed Power[a]
Intercept	178130.862	1	178130.862	1534.501	.000	.978	1534.501	1.000
Group	563.294	1	563.294	4.852	.034	.122	4.852	.572
Error	4062.935	35	116.084					

a. Computed using alpha = .05

1. Group

Measure:MEASURE_1

Group	Mean	Std. Error	95% Confidence Interval	
			Lower Bound	Upper Bound
.00	36.765	1.307	34.112	39.417
1.00	32.850	1.205	30.405	35.295

Appendix BB

Within-Subjects Factors

Measure:MEASURE_1

test	Dependent Variable
1	@1mV.1.00
2	@1mV.2.00
3	@1mV.3.00
4	@1mV.4.00

Multivariate Tests[c]

Effect		Value	F	Hypothesis df	Error df	Sig.	Partial Eta Squared	Noncent. Parameter	Observed Power[b]
test	Pillai's Trace	.013	.146[a]	3.000	33.000	.931	.013	.439	.074
	Wilks' Lambda	.987	.146[a]	3.000	33.000	.931	.013	.439	.074
	Hotelling's Trace	.013	.146[a]	3.000	33.000	.931	.013	.439	.074
	Roy's Largest Root	.013	.146[a]	3.000	33.000	.931	.013	.439	.074
test * Group	Pillai's Trace	.213	2.977[a]	3.000	33.000	.046	.213	8.932	.650
	Wilks' Lambda	.787	2.977[a]	3.000	33.000	.046	.213	8.932	.650
	Hotelling's Trace	.271	2.977[a]	3.000	33.000	.046	.213	8.932	.650
	Roy's Largest Root	.271	2.977[a]	3.000	33.000	.046	.213	8.932	.650

a. Exact statistic

b. Computed using alpha = .05

Multivariate Tests^c

Effect		Value	F	Hypothesis df	Error df	Sig.	Partial Eta Squared	Noncent. Parameter	Observed Power[b]
test	Pillai's Trace	.013	.146[a]	3.000	33.000	.931	.013	.439	.074
	Wilks' Lambda	.987	.146[a]	3.000	33.000	.931	.013	.439	.074
	Hotelling's Trace	.013	.146[a]	3.000	33.000	.931	.013	.439	.074
	Roy's Largest Root	.013	.146[a]	3.000	33.000	.931	.013	.439	.074
test * Group	Pillai's Trace	.213	2.977[a]	3.000	33.000	.046	.213	8.932	.650
	Wilks' Lambda	.787	2.977[a]	3.000	33.000	.046	.213	8.932	.650
	Hotelling's Trace	.271	2.977[a]	3.000	33.000	.046	.213	8.932	.650
	Roy's Largest Root	.271	2.977[a]	3.000	33.000	.046	.213	8.932	.650

a. Exact statistic

b. Computed using alpha = .05

c. Design: Intercept + Group
 Within Subjects Design: test

Tests of Within-Subjects Effects

Measure:MEASURE_1

Source		Type III Sum of Squares	df	Mean Square	F	Sig.	Partial Eta Squared	Noncent. Parameter	Observed Power[a]
test	Sphericity Assumed	4.859	3	1.620	.215	.886	.006	.645	.089
	Greenhouse-Geisser	4.859	2.555	1.902	.215	.857	.006	.549	.086
	Huynh-Feldt	4.859	2.852	1.704	.215	.877	.006	.613	.088
	Lower-bound	4.859	1.000	4.859	.215	.646	.006	.215	.074
test * Group	Sphericity Assumed	54.049	3	18.016	2.391	.073	.064	7.174	.584
	Greenhouse-Geisser	54.049	2.555	21.154	2.391	.083	.064	6.110	.535

	Huynh-Feldt	54.049	2.852	18.950	2.391	.076	.064	6.820	.568
	Lower-bound	54.049	1.000	54.049	2.391	.131	.064	2.391	.324
Error(test)	Sphericity Assumed	791.060	105	7.534					
	Greenhouse-Geisser	791.060	89.426	8.846					
	Huynh-Feldt	791.060	99.823	7.925					
	Lower-bound	791.060	35.000	22.602					

a. Computed using alpha = .05

3. Group * test

Measure:MEASURE_1

Group	test	Mean	Std. Error	95% Confidence Interval	
				Lower Bound	Upper Bound
.00	1	56.824	2.471	51.808	61.839
	2	55.941	2.536	50.792	61.090
	3	54.765	2.490	49.711	59.819
	4	55.765	2.745	50.193	61.337
1.00	1	49.800	2.278	45.176	54.424
	2	50.950	2.338	46.203	55.697
	3	51.150	2.295	46.490	55.810
	4	50.550	2.530	45.413	55.687

Appendix CC

Night 1

Correlations

		Sleep_Efficiency	Time_Asleep	Awakenings	Time_Awake	Avg_Time_Awake	Sleep_Latency	PSQI	ESS
Sleep_Efficiency	Pearson Correlation	1	.528**	-.327*	-.876**	-.632**	-.176	-.268	.075
	Sig. (2-tailed)		.000	.028	.000	.000	.248	.075	.626
	N	45	45	45	45	45	45	45	45
Time_Asleep	Pearson Correlation	.528**	1	.283	-.305*	-.445**	.061	-.367*	.095
	Sig. (2-tailed)	.000		.059	.042	.002	.693	.013	.536
	N	45	45	45	45	45	45	45	45
Awakenings	Pearson Correlation	-.327*	.283	1	.492**	-.293	-.040	-.192	-.173
	Sig. (2-tailed)	.028	.059		.001	.051	.793	.206	.256
	N	45	45	45	45	45	45	45	45
Time_Awake	Pearson Correlation	-.876**	-.305*	.492**	1	.441**	-.073	.145	-.101
	Sig. (2-tailed)	.000	.042	.001		.002	.634	.343	.509
	N	45	45	45	45	45	45	45	45
Avg_Time_Awake	Pearson Correlation	-.632**	-.445**	-.293	.441**	1	.201	.408**	.184
	Sig. (2-tailed)	.000	.002	.051	.002		.186	.005	.227
	N	45	45	45	45	45	45	45	45
Sleep_Latency	Pearson Correlation	-.176	.061	-.040	-.073	.201	1	-.095	.173
	Sig. (2-tailed)	.248	.693	.793	.634	.186		.537	.257
	N	45	45	45	45	45	45	45	45
PSQI	Pearson Correlation	-.268	-.367*	-.192	.145	.408**	-.095	1	.194
	Sig. (2-tailed)	.075	.013	.206	.343	.005	.537		.177
	N	45	45	45	45	45	45	50	50
ESS	Pearson Correlation	.075	.095	-.173	-.101	.184	.173	.194	1
	Sig. (2-tailed)	.626	.536	.256	.509	.227	.257	.177	
	N	45	45	45	45	45	45	50	50

**. Correlation is significant at the 0.01 level (2-tailed).
*. Correlation is significant at the 0.05 level (2-tailed).

Night 2

Correlations

		Sleep_Efficiency	Time_Asleep	Awakenings	Time_Awake	Avg_Time_Awake	Sleep_Latency	PSQI	ESS
Sleep_Efficiency	Pearson Correlation	1	.471**	-.192	-.963**	-.682**	-.457**	-.219	.116
	Sig. (2-tailed)		.003	.249	.000	.000	.004	.186	.488
	N	38	38	38	38	38	37	38	38
Time_Asleep	Pearson Correlation	.471**	1	.322*	-.263	-.527**	-.246	-.063	.122
	Sig. (2-tailed)	.003		.048	.111	.001	.142	.707	.465
	N	38	38	38	38	38	37	38	38
Awakenings	Pearson Correlation	-.192	.322*	1	.321*	-.343*	.070	-.144	.119
	Sig. (2-tailed)	.249	.048		.049	.035	.680	.387	.476
	N	38	38	38	38	38	37	38	38
Time_Awake	Pearson Correlation	-.963**	-.263	.321*	1	.571**	.488**	.237	-.125
	Sig. (2-tailed)	.000	.111	.049		.000	.002	.151	.455
	N	38	38	38	38	38	37	38	38
Avg_Time_Awake	Pearson Correlation	-.682**	-.527**	-.343*	.571**	1	.194	.350*	-.143
	Sig. (2-tailed)	.000	.001	.035	.000		.251	.031	.392
	N	38	38	38	38	38	37	38	38
Sleep_Latency	Pearson Correlation	-.457**	-.246	.070	.488**	.194	1	.159	-.263
	Sig. (2-tailed)	.004	.142	.680	.002	.251		.349	.116
	N	37	37	37	37	37	37	37	37
PSQI	Pearson Correlation	-.219	-.063	-.144	.237	.350*	.159	1	.180
	Sig. (2-tailed)	.186	.707	.387	.151	.031	.349		.267
	N	38	38	38	38	38	37	40	40
ESS	Pearson Correlation	.116	.122	.119	-.125	-.143	-.263	.180	1
	Sig. (2-tailed)	.488	.465	.476	.455	.392	.116	.267	
	N	38	38	38	38	38	37	40	40

**. Correlation is significant at the 0.01 level (2-tailed).
*. Correlation is significant at the 0.05 level (2-tailed).

Nights 1 and 2 combined

Correlations

		Sleep_Efficiency	Time_Asleep	Awakenings	Time_Awake	Avg_Time_Awake	Sleep_Latency	PSQI	ESS
Sleep_Efficiency	Pearson Correlation	1	.496**	-.233*	-.926**	-.650**	-.305**	-.250*	.103
	Sig. (2-tailed)		.000	.043	.000	.000	.008	.030	.377
	N	76	76	76	76	76	75	76	76
Time_Asleep	Pearson Correlation	.496**	1	.302**	-.285*	-.482**	-.043	-.227*	.110
	Sig. (2-tailed)	.000		.008	.013	.000	.712	.049	.346
	N	76	76	76	76	76	75	76	76
Awakenings	Pearson Correlation	-.233*	.302**	1	.381**	-.343**	.016	-.175	-.014
	Sig. (2-tailed)	.043	.008		.001	.002	.889	.132	.906
	N	76	76	76	76	76	75	76	76
Time_Awake	Pearson Correlation	-.926**	-.285*	.381**	1	.509**	.191	.199	-.120
	Sig. (2-tailed)	.000	.013	.001		.000	.101	.085	.300
	N	76	76	76	76	76	75	76	76
Avg_Time_Awake	Pearson Correlation	-.650**	-.482**	-.343**	.509**	1	.172	.385**	-.018
	Sig. (2-tailed)	.000	.000	.002	.000		.141	.001	.879
	N	76	76	76	76	76	75	76	76
Sleep_Latency	Pearson Correlation	-.305**	-.043	.016	.191	.172	1	.026	-.018
	Sig. (2-tailed)	.008	.712	.889	.101	.141		.825	.877
	N	75	75	75	75	75	75	75	75
PSQI	Pearson Correlation	-.250*	-.227*	-.175	.199	.385**	.026	1	.180
	Sig. (2-tailed)	.030	.049	.132	.085	.001	.825		.111
	N	76	76	76	76	76	75	80	80
ESS	Pearson Correlation	.103	.110	-.014	-.120	-.018	-.018	.180	1
	Sig. (2-tailed)	.377	.346	.906	.300	.879	.877	.111	
	N	76	76	76	76	76	75	80	80

**. Correlation is significant at the 0.01 level (2-tailed).
*. Correlation is significant at the 0.05 level (2-tailed).

Appendix DD

Descriptive Statistics

	Mean	Std. Deviation	N
AI	.4710	.11375	48
Gender	.5000	.50508	50
Age	22.8000	3.56285	50

Correlations

		AI	Gender	Age
Pearson Correlation	AI	1.000	-.616	.127
	Gender	-.616	1.000	-.147
	Age	.127	-.147	1.000
Sig. (1-tailed)	AI	.	.000	.196
	Gender	.000	.	.153
	Age	.196	.153	.
N	AI	48	48	48
	Gender	48	50	50
	Age	48	50	50

Model Summary[c]

Model	R	R Square	Adjusted R Square	Std. Error of the Estimate	Change Statistics					Durbin-Watson
					R Square Change	F Change	df1	df2	Sig. F Change	
1	.616[a]	.380	.366	.09057	.380	28.144	1	46	.000	

| 2 | .617[b] | .381 | .353 | .09147 | .001 | .095 | 1 | 45 | .759 | 1.849 |

a. Predictors: (Constant), Gender
b. Predictors: (Constant), Gender, Age
c. Dependent Variable: AI

ANOVA[c]

Model		Sum of Squares	df	Mean Square	F	Sig.
1	Regression	.231	1	.231	28.144	.000[a]
	Residual	.377	46	.008		
	Total	.608	47			
2	Regression	.232	2	.116	13.843	.000[b]
	Residual	.377	45	.008		
	Total	.608	47			

a. Predictors: (Constant), Gender
b. Predictors: (Constant), Gender, Age
c. Dependent Variable: AI

Coefficients[a]

Model		Unstandardized Coefficients		Standardized Coefficients	t	Sig.	95.0% Confidence Interval for B		Correlations			Collinearity Statistics	
		B	Std. Error	Beta			Lower Bound	Upper Bound	Zero-order	Partial	Part	Tolerance	VIF
1	(Constant)	.540	.018		29.224	.000	.503	.578					
	Gender	-.139	.026	-.616	-5.305	.000	-.191	-.086	-.616	-.616	-.616	1.000	1.000

2	(Constant)	.513	.090		5.686	.000	.331	.695					
	Gender	-.138	.027	-.611	-5.150	.000	-.191	-.084	-.616	-.609	-.604	.978	1.022
	Age	.001	.004	.037	.308	.759	-.006	.009	.127	.046	.036	.978	1.022

a. Dependent Variable: AI

Appendix EE

Descriptive Statistics

	Mean	Std. Deviation	N
Minus_Post_T	.0617	.06658	37
Gender	.5000	.50637	40
Age	22.5500	3.83606	40

Correlations

		Minus_Post_T	Gender	Age
Pearson Correlation	Minus_Post_T	1.000	.376	.170
	Gender	.376	1.000	-.224
	Age	.170	-.224	1.000
Sig. (1-tailed)	Minus_Post_T	.	.011	.157
	Gender	.011	.	.082
	Age	.157	.082	.
N	Minus_Post_T	37	37	37
	Gender	37	40	40
	Age	37	40	40

Model Summary[c]

Model	R	R Square	Adjusted R Square	Std. Error of the Estimate	Change Statistics	Durbin-Watson

					R Square Change	F Change	df1	df2	Sig. F Change	
1	.376a	.142	.117	.06256	.142	5.774	1	35	.022	
2	.458b	.210	.164	.06089	.068	2.946	1	34	.095	2.254

a. Predictors: (Constant), Gender

b. Predictors: (Constant), Gender, Age

c. Dependent Variable: Minus_Post_T

Coefficients[a]

Model		Unstandardized Coefficients		Standardized Coefficients	t	Sig.	95.0% Confidence Interval for B		Correlations			Collinearity Statistics	
		B	Std. Error	Beta			Lower Bound	Upper Bound	Zero-order	Partial	Part	Tolerance	VIF
1	(Constant)	.037	.015		2.538	.016	.007	.066					
	Gender	.049	.021	.376	2.403	.022	.008	.091	.376	.376	.376	1.000	1.000
2	(Constant)	-.072	.065		-1.108	.276	-.204	.060					
	Gender	.057	.021	.437	2.791	.009	.016	.099	.376	.432	.425	.950	1.053
	Age	.005	.003	.268	1.716	.095	-.001	.010	.170	.282	.262	.950	1.053

a. Dependent Variable: Minus_Post_T

Appendix FF

Descriptive Statistics

	Mean	Std. Deviation	N
AI	.6245	.06944	38
LogPP3_tot	-.4939	.40426	39
LogPP10_total	.0348	.22728	39

Correlations

		AI	LogPP3_tot	LogPP10_total
Pearson Correlation	AI	1.000	-.504	-.536
	LogPP3_tot	-.504	1.000	.138
	LogPP10_total	-.536	.138	1.000
Sig. (1-tailed)	AI	.	.001	.000
	LogPP3_tot	.001	.	.201
	LogPP10_total	.000	.201	.
N	AI	38	37	37
	LogPP3_tot	37	39	39
	LogPP10_total	37	39	39

Model Summary[c]

Model	R	R Square	Adjusted R Square	Std. Error of the Estimate	Change Statistics					Durbin-Watson
					R Square Change	F Change	df1	df2	Sig. F Change	
1	.504[a]	.254	.233	.06083	.254	11.913	1	35	.001	

| 2 | .690[b] | .476 | .445 | .05172 | .222 | 14.409 | 1 | 34 | .001 | 2.273 |

a. Predictors: (Constant), LogPP3_tot
b. Predictors: (Constant), LogPP3_tot, LogPP10_total
c. Dependent Variable: AI

ANOVA[c]

Model		Sum of Squares	df	Mean Square	F	Sig.
1	Regression	.044	1	.044	11.913	.001[a]
	Residual	.130	35	.004		
	Total	.174	36			
2	Regression	.083	2	.041	15.443	.000[b]
	Residual	.091	34	.003		
	Total	.174	36			

a. Predictors: (Constant), LogPP3_tot
b. Predictors: (Constant), LogPP3_tot, LogPP10_total
c. Dependent Variable: AI

Coefficients[a]

Model		Unstandardized Coefficients		Standardized Coefficients	t	Sig.	95.0% Confidence Interval for B		Correlations			Collinearity Statistics	
		B	Std. Error	Beta			Lower Bound	Upper Bound	Zero-order	Partial	Part	Tolerance	VIF
1	(Constant)	.582	.016		36.542	.000	.549	.614					
	LogPP3_tot	-.087	.025	-.504	-3.452	.001	-.137	-.036	-.504	-.504	-.504	1.000	1.000
2	(Constant)	.592	.014		42.854	.000	.564	.620					
	LogPP3_tot	-.075	.022	-.438	-3.497	.001	-.119	-.032	-.504	-.514	-.434	.981	1.019

Model Summary[c]

Model	R	R Square	Adjusted R Square	Std. Error of the Estimate	Change Statistics					Durbin-Watson
					R Square Change	F Change	df1	df2	Sig. F Change	
1	.504[a]	.254	.233	.06083	.254	11.913	1	35	.001	
2	.690[b]	.476	.445	.05172	.222	14.409	1	34	.001	2.273

a. Predictors: (Constant), LogPP3_tot

b. Predictors: (Constant), LogPP3_tot, LogPP10_total

| | LogPP10_total | -.145 | .038 | -.476 | -3.796 | .001 | -.223 | -.068 | -.536 | -.546 | -.471 | .981 | 1.019 |

a. Dependent Variable: AI

Appendix GG

Descriptive Statistics

	Mean	Std. Deviation	N
AI	.6133	.06691	20
LogPP3_tot	-.3804	.39604	20
LogPP10_total	.0015	.23597	20

Correlations

		AI	LogPP3_tot	LogPP10_total
Pearson Correlation	AI	1.000	-.344	-.647
	LogPP3_tot	-.344	1.000	.262
	LogPP10_total	-.647	.262	1.000
Sig. (1-tailed)	AI	.	.069	.001
	LogPP3_tot	.069	.	.132
	LogPP10_total	.001	.132	.
N	AI	20	20	20
	LogPP3_tot	20	20	20
	LogPP10_total	20	20	20

Model Summary[c]

Model	R	R Square	Adjusted R Square	Std. Error of the Estimate	Change Statistics					Durbin-Watson
					R Square Change	F Change	df1	df2	Sig. F Change	
1	.344[a]	.119	.070	.06454	.119	2.420	1	18	.137	

| 2 | .672[b] | .451 | .386 | .05241 | .332 | 10.295 | 1 | 17 | .005 | 1.785 |

a. Predictors: (Constant), LogPP3_tot

b. Predictors: (Constant), LogPP3_tot, LogPP10_total

c. Dependent Variable: AI

ANOVA[c]

Model		Sum of Squares	df	Mean Square	F	Sig.
1	Regression	.010	1	.010	2.420	.137[a]
	Residual	.075	18	.004		
	Total	.085	19			
2	Regression	.038	2	.019	6.983	.006[b]
	Residual	.047	17	.003		
	Total	.085	19			

a. Predictors: (Constant), LogPP3_tot

b. Predictors: (Constant), LogPP3_tot, LogPP10_total

c. Dependent Variable: AI

Coefficients[a]

Model		Unstandardized Coefficients		Standardized Coefficients	t	Sig.	95.0% Confidence Interval for B		Correlations			Collinearity Statistics	
		B	Std. Error	Beta			Lower Bound	Upper Bound	Zero-order	Partial	Part	Tolerance	VIF
1	(Constant)	.591	.020		29.172	.000	.549	.634					
	LogPP3_tot	-.058	.037	-.344	-1.556	.137	-.137	.020	-.344	-.344	-.344	1.000	1.000

2	(Constant)	.601	.017		35.871	.000	.566	.637					
	LogPP3_tot	-.032	.031	-.188	-1.007	.328	-.098	.035	-.344	-.237	-.181	.931	1.074
	LogPP10_total	-.169	.053	-.598	-3.209	.005	-.281	-.058	-.647	-.614	-.577	.931	1.074

a. Dependent Variable: AI

Appendix HH

Descriptive Statistics

	Mean	Std. Deviation	N
AI	.4594	.13888	49
rMT	43.9388	7.80066	49
@1mV	51.4898	10.01899	49
aMT	33.4490	5.82044	49

Correlations

		AI	rMT	@1mV	aMT
Pearson Correlation	AI	1.000	.253	.019	.144
	rMT	.253	1.000	.798	.829
	@1mV	.019	.798	1.000	.824
	aMT	.144	.829	.824	1.000
Sig. (1-tailed)	AI	.	.042	.449	.164
	rMT	.042	.	.000	.000
	@1mV	.449	.000	.	.000
	aMT	.164	.000	.000	.
N	AI	49	48	48	48
	rMT	48	49	49	49
	@1mV	48	49	49	49
	aMT	48	49	49	49

Model Summary[d]

Model	R	R Square	Adjusted R Square	Std. Error of the Estimate	Change Statistics					Durbin-Watson
					R Square Change	F Change	df1	df2	Sig. F Change	
1	.253[a]	.064	.043	.13583	.064	3.136	1	46	.083	
2	.394[b]	.156	.118	.13043	.092	4.892	1	45	.032	
3	.396[c]	.157	.099	.13181	.001	.060	1	44	.808	2.239

a. Predictors: (Constant), rMT
b. Predictors: (Constant), rMT, @1mV
c. Predictors: (Constant), rMT, @1mV, aMT
d. Dependent Variable: AI

Coefficients[a]

Model	Unstandardized Coefficients		Standardized Coefficients	t	Sig.	95.0% Confidence Interval for B		Correlations			Collinearity Statistics	
	B	Std. Error	Beta			Lower Bound	Upper Bound	Zero-order	Partial	Part	Tolerance	VIF
1 (Constant)	.262	.113		2.310	.025	.034	.490					
rMT	.004	.003	.253	1.771	.083	-.001	.010	.253	.253	.253	1.000	1.000

2	(Constant)	.307	.111		2.771	.008	.084	.530						
	rMT	.012	.004	.654	2.876	.006	.003	.020	.253	.394	.394		.363	2.753
	@1mV	-.007	.003	-.503	-2.212	.032	-.013	-.001	.019	-.313	-.303		.363	2.753
3	(Constant)	.299	.116		2.578	.013	.065	.533						
	rMT	.011	.005	.621	2.337	.024	.002	.021	.253	.332	.324		.271	3.684
	@1mV	-.007	.004	-.534	-2.035	.048	-.015	.000	.019	-.293	-.282		.279	3.588
	aMT	.002	.007	.069	.245	.808	-.012	.015	.144	.037	.034		.240	4.175

a. Dependent Variable: AI

Descriptive Statistics

	Mean	Std. Deviation	N
AI_pos_0	.5482	.10808	49
rMT	43.9388	7.80066	49
@1mV	51.4898	10.01899	49
aMT	33.4490	5.82044	49

Correlations

		AI_pos_0	rMT	@1mV	aMT
Pearson Correlation	AI_pos_0	1.000	.188	-.043	.085
	rMT	.188	1.000	.798	.829
	@1mV	-.043	.798	1.000	.824
	aMT	.085	.829	.824	1.000

Sig. (1-tailed)	AI_pos_0	.	.100	.387	.283
	rMT	.100	.	.000	.000
	@1mV	.387	.000	.	.000
	aMT	.283	.000	.000	.
N	AI_pos_0	49	48	48	48
	rMT	48	49	49	49
	@1mV	48	49	49	49
	aMT	48	49	49	49

Model Summary[d]

Model	R	R Square	Adjusted R Square	Std. Error of the Estimate	Change Statistics					Durbin-Watson
					R Square Change	F Change	df1	df2	Sig. F Change	
1	.188[a]	.035	.014	.10730	.035	1.689	1	46	.200	
2	.371[b]	.138	.099	.10257	.102	5.333	1	45	.026	

| 3 | .372[c] | .139 | .080 | .10368 | .001 | .048 | 1 | 44 | .827 | 2.108 |

a. Predictors: (Constant), rMT

b. Predictors: (Constant), rMT, @1mV

c. Predictors: (Constant), rMT, @1mV, aMT

d. Dependent Variable: AI_pos_0

Coefficients[a]

Model		Unstandardized Coefficients		Standardized Coefficients	t	Sig.	95.0% Confidence Interval for B		Correlations			Collinearity Statistics	
		B	Std. Error	Beta			Lower Bound	Upper Bound	Zero-order	Partial	Part	Tolerance	VIF
1	(Constant)	.434	.090		4.845	.000	.253	.614					
	rMT	.003	.002	.188	1.300	.200	-.001	.007	.188	.188	.188	1.000	1.000
2	(Constant)	.471	.087		5.406	.000	.295	.646					
	rMT	.008	.003	.611	2.662	.011	.002	.015	.188	.369	.369	.363	2.753
	@1mV	-.006	.002	-.530	-2.309	.026	-.011	-.001	-.043	-.326	-.320	.363	2.753
3	(Constant)	.465	.091		5.097	.000	.281	.649					
	rMT	.008	.004	.582	2.166	.036	.001	.016	.188	.310	.303	.271	3.684
	@1mV	-.006	.003	-.559	-2.107	.041	-.012	.000	-.043	-.303	-.295	.279	3.588

| aMT | .001 | .005 | .063 | .220 | .827 | -.010 | .012 | .085 | .033 | .031 | .240 | 4.175 |

a. Dependent Variable: Al_pos_0

Descriptive Statistics

	Mean	Std. Deviation	N
Al_neg_1	.3701	.19076	49
rMT	43.9388	7.80066	49
@1mV	51.4898	10.01899	49
aMT	33.4490	5.82044	49

Correlations

		Al_neg_1	rMT	@1mV	aMT
Pearson Correlation	Al_neg_1	1.000	.261	.052	.162
	rMT	.261	1.000	.798	.829
	@1mV	.052	.798	1.000	.824
	aMT	.162	.829	.824	1.000
Sig. (1-tailed)	Al_neg_1	.	.037	.363	.135
	rMT	.037	.	.000	.000
	@1mV	.363	.000	.	.000
	aMT	.135	.000	.000	.
N	Al_neg_1	49	48	48	48
	rMT	48	49	49	49
	@1mV	48	49	49	49
	aMT	48	49	49	49

Model Summary[d]

Model	R	R Square	Adjusted R Square	Std. Error of the Estimate	Change Statistics					Durbin-Watson
					R Square Change	F Change	df1	df2	Sig. F Change	
1	.261[a]	.068	.048	.18613	.068	3.366	1	46	.073	
2	.368[b]	.136	.097	.18124	.068	3.516	1	45	.067	
3	.370[c]	.137	.078	.18318	.001	.052	1	44	.820	2.329

a. Predictors: (Constant), rMT
b. Predictors: (Constant), rMT, @1mV
c. Predictors: (Constant), rMT, @1mV, aMT
d. Dependent Variable: AI_neg_1

Coefficients[a]

Model	Unstandardized Coefficients		Standardized Coefficients	t	Sig.	95.0% Confidence Interval for B		Correlations			Collinearity Statistics	
	B	Std. Error	Beta			Lower Bound	Upper Bound	Zero-order	Partial	Part	Tolerance	VIF

1	(Constant)	.090	.155		.577	.567	-.223	.402					
	rMT	.006	.003	.261	1.835	.073	-.001	.013	.261	.261	.261	1.000	1.000
2	(Constant)	.143	.154		.927	.359	-.167	.452					
	rMT	.015	.006	.605	2.632	.012	.003	.026	.261	.365	.365	.363	2.753
	@1mV	-.008	.004	-.431	-1.875	.067	-.017	.001	.052	-.269	-.260	.363	2.753
3	(Constant)	.133	.161		.823	.415	-.192	.458					
	rMT	.014	.007	.574	2.136	.038	.001	.027	.261	.307	.299	.271	3.684
	@1mV	-.009	.005	-.460	-1.735	.090	-.019	.001	.052	-.253	-.243	.279	3.588
	aMT	.002	.009	.065	.229	.820	-.017	.021	.162	.034	.032	.240	4.175

a. Dependent Variable: AI_neg_1

Appendix II

Descriptive Statistics

	Mean	Std. Deviation	N
AI_pos_0	.6525	.08348	20
Avg_Time_Awake	3.9789	2.92090	19
Awakenings	17.7895	8.23663	19
Sleep_Efficiency	84.7216	7.49921	19

Correlations

		AI_pos_0	Avg_Time_Awake	Awakenings	Sleep_Efficiency
Pearson Correlation	AI_pos_0	1.000	-.236	-.346	.368
	Avg_Time_Awake	-.236	1.000	-.428	-.652
	Awakenings	-.346	-.428	1.000	-.208
	Sleep_Efficiency	.368	-.652	-.208	1.000
Sig. (1-tailed)	AI_pos_0	.	.165	.073	.061
	Avg_Time_Awake	.165	.	.034	.001
	Awakenings	.073	.034	.	.196
	Sleep_Efficiency	.061	.001	.196	.
N	AI_pos_0	20	19	19	19
	Avg_Time_Awake	19	19	19	19
	Awakenings	19	19	19	19
	Sleep_Efficiency	19	19	19	19

Model Summary[d]

Model	R	R Square	Adjusted R Square	Std. Error of the Estimate	Change Statistics					Durbin-Watson
					R Square Change	F Change	df1	df2	Sig. F Change	
1	.236[a]	.056	.000	.08348	.056	1.002	1	17	.331	
2	.548[b]	.300	.213	.07407	.245	5.593	1	16	.031	
3	.557[c]	.310	.172	.07596	.010	.212	1	15	.652	2.973

a. Predictors: (Constant), Avg_Time_Awake

b. Predictors: (Constant), Avg_Time_Awake, Awakenings

c. Predictors: (Constant), Avg_Time_Awake, Awakenings, Sleep_Efficiency

d. Dependent Variable: AI_pos_0

ANOVA[d]

Model		Sum of Squares	df	Mean Square	F	Sig.
1	Regression	.007	1	.007	1.002	.331[a]
	Residual	.118	17	.007		
	Total	.125	18			
2	Regression	.038	2	.019	3.433	.057[b]
	Residual	.088	16	.005		
	Total	.125	18			
3	Regression	.039	3	.013	2.247	.125[c]
	Residual	.087	15	.006		
	Total	.125	18			

a. Predictors: (Constant), Avg_Time_Awake

b. Predictors: (Constant), Avg_Time_Awake, Awakenings

c. Predictors: (Constant), Avg_Time_Awake, Awakenings, Sleep_Efficiency

d. Dependent Variable: AI_pos_0

Coefficients[a]

Model	Unstandardized Coefficients		Standardized Coefficients	t	Sig.	95.0% Confidence Interval for B		Correlations			Collinearity Statistics	
	B	Std. Error	Beta			Lower Bound	Upper Bound	Zero-order	Partial	Part	Tolerance	VIF
1 (Constant)	.679	.033		20.621	.000	.610	.749					
Avg_Time_Awake	-.007	.007	-.236	-1.001	.331	-.021	.007	-.236	-.236	-.236	1.000	1.000
2 (Constant)	.805	.061		13.297	.000	.676	.933					
Avg_Time_Awake	-.013	.007	-.470	-2.032	.059	-.027	.001	-.236	-.453	-.425	.817	1.224
Awakenings	-.006	.002	-.547	-2.365	.031	-.011	-.001	-.346	-.509	-.495	.817	1.224
3 (Constant)	1.018	.468		2.176	.046	.021	2.015					
Avg_Time_Awake	-.018	.012	-.638	-1.467	.163	-.045	.008	-.236	-.354	-.315	.243	4.111
Awakenings	-.007	.003	-.657	-1.950	.070	-.014	.001	-.346	-.450	-.418	.404	2.473
Sleep_Efficiency	-.002	.004	-.185	-.460	.652	-.012	.007	.368	-.118	-.099	.285	3.510

a. Dependent Variable: AI_pos_0

Appendix JJ

Descriptive Statistics

	Mean	Std. Deviation	N
AI_neg_1	.5695	.09055	20
Avg_Time_Awake	3.6729	1.97722	18
Awakenings	22.0556	12.37869	18
Sleep_Efficiency	85.2750	7.53149	18

Correlations

		AI_neg_1	Avg_Time_Awake	Awakenings	Sleep_Efficiency
Pearson Correlation	AI_neg_1	1.000	.480	.101	-.160
	Avg_Time_Awake	.480	1.000	-.401	-.234
	Awakenings	.101	-.401	1.000	-.522
	Sleep_Efficiency	-.160	-.234	-.522	1.000
Sig. (1-tailed)	AI_neg_1	.	.022	.345	.263
	Avg_Time_Awake	.022	.	.050	.175
	Awakenings	.345	.050	.	.013
	Sleep_Efficiency	.263	.175	.013	.
N	AI_neg_1	20	18	18	18
	Avg_Time_Awake	18	18	18	18
	Awakenings	18	18	18	18
	Sleep_Efficiency	18	18	18	18

Model Summary[d]

Model	R	R Square	Adjusted R Square	Std. Error of the Estimate	Change Statistics					Durbin-Watson
					R Square Change	F Change	df1	df2	Sig. F Change	
1	.480[a]	.230	.182	.08188	.230	4.792	1	16	.044	
2	.577[b]	.333	.244	.07873	.103	2.306	1	15	.150	
3	.624[c]	.390	.259	.07796	.057	1.299	1	14	.274	1.889

a. Predictors: (Constant), Avg_Time_Awake

b. Predictors: (Constant), Avg_Time_Awake, Awakenings

c. Predictors: (Constant), Avg_Time_Awake, Awakenings, Sleep_Efficiency

d. Dependent Variable: AI_neg_1

ANOVA[d]

Model		Sum of Squares	df	Mean Square	F	Sig.
1	Regression	.032	1	.032	4.792	.044[a]
	Residual	.107	16	.007		
	Total	.139	17			
2	Regression	.046	2	.023	3.744	.048[b]
	Residual	.093	15	.006		
	Total	.139	17			
3	Regression	.054	3	.018	2.979	.068[c]
	Residual	.085	14	.006		
	Total	.139	17			

a. Predictors: (Constant), Avg_Time_Awake

b. Predictors: (Constant), Avg_Time_Awake, Awakenings

c. Predictors: (Constant), Avg_Time_Awake, Awakenings, Sleep_Efficiency

ANOVA[d]

Model		Sum of Squares	df	Mean Square	F	Sig.
1	Regression	.032	1	.032	4.792	.044[a]
	Residual	.107	16	.007		
	Total	.139	17			
2	Regression	.046	2	.023	3.744	.048[b]
	Residual	.093	15	.006		
	Total	.139	17			
3	Regression	.054	3	.018	2.979	.068[c]
	Residual	.085	14	.006		
	Total	.139	17			

a. Predictors: (Constant), Avg_Time_Awake

b. Predictors: (Constant), Avg_Time_Awake, Awakenings

c. Predictors: (Constant), Avg_Time_Awake, Awakenings, Sleep_Efficiency

d. Dependent Variable: AI_neg_1

Coefficients[a]

Model		Unstandardized Coefficients		Standardized Coefficients	t	Sig.	95.0% Confidence Interval for B		Correlations			Collinearity Statistics	
		B	Std. Error	Beta			Lower Bound	Upper Bound	Zero-order	Partial	Part	Tolerance	VIF
1	(Constant)	.489	.042		11.739	.000	.400	.577					
	Avg_Time_Awake	.022	.010	.480	2.189	.044	.001	.043	.480	.480	.480	1.000	1.000
2	(Constant)	.409	.066		6.181	.000	.268	.550					
	Avg_Time_Awake	.028	.011	.620	2.694	.017	.006	.051	.480	.571	.568	.839	1.191

	Awakenings	.003	.002	.349	1.518	.150	-.001	.006	.101	.365	.320	.839	1.191
3	(Constant)	-.008	.372		-.022	.983	-.806	.789					
	Avg_Time_Awake	.037	.013	.799	2.888	.012	.009	.064	.480	.611	.603	.570	1.754
	Awakenings	.004	.002	.598	1.896	.079	-.001	.009	.101	.452	.396	.439	2.278
	Sleep_Efficiency	.004	.004	.338	1.140	.274	-.004	.012	-.160	.291	.238	.494	2.023

a. Dependent Variable: AI_neg_1

Appendix KK

Descriptive Statistics

	Mean	Std. Deviation	N
AI_neg_1	.5958	.08440	19
Avg_Time_Awake	3.6729	1.97722	18
Awakenings	22.0556	12.37869	18
Sleep_Efficiency	85.2750	7.53149	18

Model Summary[d]

Model	R	R Square	Adjusted R Square	Std. Error of the Estimate	Change Statistics					Durbin-Watson
					R Square Change	F Change	df1	df2	Sig. F Change	
1	.279[a]	.078	.017	.08369	.078	1.271	1	15	.277	
2	.602[b]	.363	.272	.07202	.285	6.254	1	14	.025	
3	.607[c]	.369	.223	.07440	.006	.121	1	13	.734	1.941

a. Predictors: (Constant), Avg_Time_Awake

b. Predictors: (Constant), Avg_Time_Awake, Awakenings

c. Predictors: (Constant), Avg_Time_Awake, Awakenings, Sleep_Efficiency

d. Dependent Variable: AI_neg_1

ANOVA[d]

Model		Sum of Squares	df	Mean Square	F	Sig.
1	Regression	.009	1	.009	1.271	.277[a]
	Residual	.105	15	.007		

			B	Std. Error	Beta	t	Sig.	Lower Bound	Upper Bound	Zero-order	Partial	Part	Tolerance	VIF
		Total	.114	16										
2		Regression	.041	2	.021	3.985	.043[b]							
		Residual	.073	14	.005									
		Total	.114	16										
3		Regression	.042	3	.014	2.530	.103[c]							
		Residual	.072	13	.006									
		Total	.114	16										

a. Predictors: (Constant), Avg_Time_Awake

b. Predictors: (Constant), Avg_Time_Awake, Awakenings

c. Predictors: (Constant), Avg_Time_Awake, Awakenings, Sleep_Efficiency

d. Dependent Variable: AI_neg_1

Coefficients[a]

Model		Unstandardized Coefficients		Standardized Coefficients	t	Sig.	95.0% Confidence Interval for B		Correlations			Collinearity Statistics	
		B	Std. Error	Beta			Lower Bound	Upper Bound	Zero-order	Partial	Part	Tolerance	VIF
1	(Constant)	.552	.044		12.589	.000	.459	.645					
	Avg_Time_Awake	.012	.011	.279	1.127	.277	-.011	.034	.279	.279	.279	1.000	1.000
2	(Constant)	.428	.062		6.862	.000	.294	.562					
	Avg_Time_Awake	.022	.010	.513	2.202	.045	.001	.043	.279	.507	.470	.839	1.191
	Awakenings	.004	.002	.582	2.501	.025	.001	.007	.377	.556	.534	.839	1.191
3	(Constant)	.303	.366		.828	.423	-.487	1.093					

Avg_Time_Awake	.024	.012		.570	1.954	.073	-.003	.051	.279	.476	.431	.570	1.754
Awakenings	.005	.002		.662	1.991	.068	.000	.009	.377	.483	.439	.439	2.278
Sleep_Efficiency	.001	.004		.109	.348	.734	-.006	.009	-.370	.096	.077	.494	2.023

a. Dependent Variable: AI_neg_1

Appendix LL

Descriptive Statistics

	Mean	Std. Deviation	N
Minus_Post_C	.0299	.05605	19
Avg_Time_Awake	4.4860	4.72520	20
Awakenings	17.9500	7.49368	20
Sleep_Efficiency	84.8055	11.14568	20

Model Summary[d]

Model	R	R Square	Adjusted R Square	Std. Error of the Estimate	Change Statistics					Durbin-Watson
					R Square Change	F Change	df1	df2	Sig. F Change	
1	.312[a]	.097	.044	.05481	.097	1.827	1	17	.194	
2	.682[b]	.465	.398	.04349	.368	10.998	1	16	.004	
3	.802[c]	.644	.573	.03664	.179	7.544	1	15	.015	1.872

a. Predictors: (Constant), Avg_Time_Awake

b. Predictors: (Constant), Avg_Time_Awake, Awakenings

c. Predictors: (Constant), Avg_Time_Awake, Awakenings, Sleep_Efficiency

d. Dependent Variable: Minus_Post_C

ANOVA[d]

Model		Sum of Squares	df	Mean Square	F	Sig.
1	Regression	.005	1	.005	1.827	.194[a]
	Residual	.051	17	.003		

			.057	18			
2	Regression		.026	2	.013	6.949	.007[b]
	Residual		.030	16	.002		
	Total		.057	18			
3	Regression		.036	3	.012	9.043	.001[c]
	Residual		.020	15	.001		
	Total		.057	18			

a. Predictors: (Constant), Avg_Time_Awake

b. Predictors: (Constant), Avg_Time_Awake, Awakenings

c. Predictors: (Constant), Avg_Time_Awake, Awakenings, Sleep_Efficiency

d. Dependent Variable: Minus_Post_C

Coefficients[a]

Model		Unstandardized Coefficients		Standardized Coefficients	t	Sig.	Correlations			Collinearity Statistics	
		B	Std. Error	Beta			Zero-order	Partial	Part	Tolerance	VIF
1	(Constant)	.046	.018		2.647	.017					
	Avg_Time_Awake	-.004	.003	-.312	-1.352	.194	-.312	-.312	-.312	1.000	1.000
2	(Constant)	.150	.034		4.387	.000					
	Avg_Time_Awake	-.007	.002	-.583	-2.911	.010	-.312	-.588	-.532	.833	1.201
	Awakenings	-.005	.001	-.665	-3.316	.004	-.426	-.638	-.606	.833	1.201
3	(Constant)	-.279	.159		-1.756	.100					

Avg_Time_Awake	.002	.004	.195	.591	.563	-.312	.151	.091	.218	4.585
Awakenings	-.003	.001	-.411	-2.136	.050	-.426	-.483	-.329	.641	1.560
Sleep_Efficiency	.004	.002	.829	2.747	.015	.639	.578	.423	.260	3.841

a. Dependent Variable: Minus_Post_C

Appendix MM

```
[DataSet2] C:\Documents and Settings\mborich\Desktop\PASW_Sleep\AI_triallonly.sav
```

Within-Subjects Factors

Measure:MEASURE_1

Assessment	Dependent Variable
1	AI_comp.1.00
2	AI_comp.2.00
3	AI_comp.3.00
4	AI_comp.4.00

Multivariate Tests[c]

Effect		Value	F	Hypothesis df	Error df	Sig.	Partial Eta Squared	Noncent. Parameter	Observed Power[b]
Assessment	Pillai's Trace	.356	7.733[a]	3.000	42.000	.000	.356	23.199	.981
	Wilks' Lambda	.644	7.733[a]	3.000	42.000	.000	.356	23.199	.981
	Hotelling's Trace	.552	7.733[a]	3.000	42.000	.000	.356	23.199	.981
	Roy's Largest Root	.552	7.733[a]	3.000	42.000	.000	.356	23.199	.981
Assessment * Track_Train	Pillai's Trace	.099	1.538[a]	3.000	42.000	.219	.099	4.613	.376
	Wilks' Lambda	.901	1.538[a]	3.000	42.000	.219	.099	4.613	.376

	Hotelling's Trace	.110	1.538[a]	3.000	42.000	.219	.099	4.613	.376
	Roy's Largest Root	.110	1.538[a]	3.000	42.000	.219	.099	4.613	.376

a. Exact statistic

b. Computed using alpha = .05

c. Design: Intercept + Track_Train
 Within Subjects Design: Assessment

Mauchly's Test of Sphericity[b]

Measure:MEASURE_1

Within Subjects Effect	Mauchly's W	Approx. Chi-Square	df	Sig.	Epsilon[a]		
					Greenhouse-Geisser	Huynh-Feldt	Lower-bound
Assessment	.314	49.453	5	.000	.570	.604	.333

Tests the null hypothesis that the error covariance matrix of the orthonormalized transformed dependent variables is proportional to an identity matrix.

a. May be used to adjust the degrees of freedom for the averaged tests of significance. Corrected tests are displayed in the Tests of Within-Subjects Effects table.

b. Design: Intercept + Track_Train
 Within Subjects Design: Assessment

Tests of Within-Subjects Effects

Measure:MEASURE_1

Source		Type III Sum of Squares	df	Mean Square	F	Sig.	Partial Eta Squared	Noncent. Parameter	Observed Power[a]
Assessment	Sphericity Assumed	.437	3	.146	14.211	.000	.244	42.633	1.000
	Greenhouse-Geisser	.437	1.710	.255	14.211	.000	.244	24.300	.996
	Huynh-Feldt	.437	1.813	.241	14.211	.000	.244	25.760	.997
	Lower-bound	.437	1.000	.437	14.211	.000	.244	14.211	.958
Assessment * Track_Train	Sphericity Assumed	.067	3	.022	2.189	.092	.047	6.567	.546
	Greenhouse-Geisser	.067	1.710	.039	2.189	.126	.047	3.743	.401
	Huynh-Feldt	.067	1.813	.037	2.189	.123	.047	3.968	.414
	Lower-bound	.067	1.000	.067	2.189	.146	.047	2.189	.304
Error(Assessment)	Sphericity Assumed	1.352	132	.010					
	Greenhouse-Geisser	1.352	75.238	.018					
	Huynh-Feldt	1.352	79.757	.017					
	Lower-bound	1.352	44.000	.031					

a. Computed using alpha = .05

Tests of Between-Subjects Effects

Measure:MEASURE_1

Transformed Variable:Average

Source	Type III Sum of Squares	df	Mean Square	F	Sig.	Partial Eta Squared	Noncent. Parameter	Observed Power[a]
Intercept	39.693	1	39.693	1347.018	.000	.968	1347.018	1.000
Track_Train	.001	1	.001	.034	.854	.001	.034	.054
Error	1.297	44	.029					

a. Computed using alpha = .05

3. Track_Train * Assessment

Measure:MEASURE_1

Track_Train	Assessment	Mean	Std. Error	95% Confidence Interval	
				Lower Bound	Upper Bound
.00	1	.513	.066	.381	.646
	2	.573	.028	.517	.628
	3	.622	.032	.558	.686
	4	.622	.024	.573	.671
1.00	1	.449	.032	.383	.514
	2	.637	.014	.610	.665
	3	.613	.016	.582	.645
	4	.654	.012	.630	.678

Within-Subjects Factors

Measure:MEASURE_1

Assessment	Dependent Variable
1	AI_incomp.1.00
2	AI_incomp.2.00
3	AI_incomp.3.00
4	AI_incomp.4.00

Multivariate Tests[c]

Effect		Value	F	Hypothesis df	Error df	Sig.	Partial Eta Squared	Noncent. Parameter	Observed Power[b]
Assessment	Pillai's Trace	.519	14.768[a]	3.000	41.000	.000	.519	44.305	1.000
	Wilks' Lambda	.481	14.768[a]	3.000	41.000	.000	.519	44.305	1.000
	Hotelling's Trace	1.081	14.768[a]	3.000	41.000	.000	.519	44.305	1.000
	Roy's Largest Root	1.081	14.768[a]	3.000	41.000	.000	.519	44.305	1.000
Assessment * Track_Train	Pillai's Trace	.017	.233[a]	3.000	41.000	.873	.017	.698	.090
	Wilks' Lambda	.983	.233[a]	3.000	41.000	.873	.017	.698	.090
	Hotelling's Trace	.017	.233[a]	3.000	41.000	.873	.017	.698	.090

| | Roy's Largest Root | .017 | .233[a] | 3.000 | 41.000 | .873 | .017 | .698 | .090 |

a. Exact statistic

b. Computed using alpha = .05

c. Design: Intercept + Track_Train
 Within Subjects Design: Assessment

Tests of Within-Subjects Effects

Measure:MEASURE_1

Source		Type III Sum of Squares	df	Mean Square	F	Sig.	Partial Eta Squared	Noncent. Parameter	Observed Power[a]
Assessment	Sphericity Assumed	3.214	3	1.071	32.302	.000	.429	96.905	1.000
	Greenhouse-Geisser	3.214	1.811	1.775	32.302	.000	.429	58.501	1.000
	Huynh-Feldt	3.214	1.930	1.665	32.302	.000	.429	62.345	1.000
	Lower-bound	3.214	1.000	3.214	32.302	.000	.429	32.302	1.000
Assessment * Track_Train	Sphericity Assumed	.018	3	.006	.183	.908	.004	.550	.083
	Greenhouse-Geisser	.018	1.811	.010	.183	.812	.004	.332	.076
	Huynh-Feldt	.018	1.930	.009	.183	.825	.004	.354	.077
	Lower-bound	.018	1.000	.018	.183	.671	.004	.183	.070
Error(Assessment)	Sphericity Assumed	4.279	129	.033					
	Greenhouse-Geisser	4.279	77.876	.055					

	Huynh-Feldt	4.279	82.994	.052				
	Lower-bound	4.279	43.000	.100				

a. Computed using alpha = .05

Tests of Between-Subjects Effects

Measure:MEASURE_1

Transformed Variable:Average

Source	Type III Sum of Squares	df	Mean Square	F	Sig.	Partial Eta Squared	Noncent. Parameter	Observed Power[a]
Intercept	19.257	1	19.257	142.111	.000	.768	142.111	1.000
Track_Train	.076	1	.076	.559	.459	.013	.559	.113
Error	5.827	43	.136					

a. Computed using alpha = .05

3. Track_Train * Assessment

Measure:MEASURE_1

Track_Train	Assessment	Mean	Std. Error	95% Confidence Interval	
				Lower Bound	Upper Bound
.00	1	.172	.130	-.090	.433
	2	.540	.077	.384	.696
	3	.515	.062	.389	.641
	4	.592	.052	.488	.696
1.00	1	.084	.060	-.037	.206
	2	.476	.036	.403	.549
	3	.500	.029	.442	.559

3. Track_Train * Assessment

Measure:MEASURE_1

Track_Train	Assessment	Mean	Std. Error	95% Confidence Interval	
				Lower Bound	Upper Bound
.00	1	.172	.130	-.090	.433
	2	.540	.077	.384	.696
	3	.515	.062	.389	.641
	4	.592	.052	.488	.696
	1	.084	.060	-.037	.206
	2	.476	.036	.403	.549
	3	.500	.029	.442	.559
	4	.543	.024	.495	.592

[DataSet4] C:\Documents and Settings\mborich\Desktop\PASW_Sleep\Tracking_mean_notrial1.sav

Within-Subjects Factors

Measure:MEASURE_1

Assessment	Dependent Variable
1	AI_comp.1.00
2	AI_comp.2.00
3	AI_comp.3.00
4	AI_comp.4.00

Multivariate Tests [c]

Effect		Value	F	Hypothesis df	Error df	Sig.	Partial Eta Squared	Noncent. Parameter	Observed Power [b]
Assessment	Pillai's Trace	.641	24.984[a]	3.000	42.000	.000	.641	74.953	1.000
	Wilks' Lambda	.359	24.984[a]	3.000	42.000	.000	.641	74.953	1.000
	Hotelling's Trace	1.785	24.984[a]	3.000	42.000	.000	.641	74.953	1.000
	Roy's Largest Root	1.785	24.984[a]	3.000	42.000	.000	.641	74.953	1.000
Assessment * Track_Train	Pillai's Trace	.128	2.046[a]	3.000	42.000	.122	.128	6.138	.487
	Wilks' Lambda	.872	2.046[a]	3.000	42.000	.122	.128	6.138	.487
	Hotelling's Trace	.146	2.046[a]	3.000	42.000	.122	.128	6.138	.487
	Roy's Largest Root	.146	2.046[a]	3.000	42.000	.122	.128	6.138	.487

a. Exact statistic

b. Computed using alpha = .05

c. Design: Intercept + Track_Train
Within Subjects Design: Assessment

Tests of Within-Subjects Effects

Measure:MEASURE_1

Source		Type III Sum of Squares	df	Mean Square	F	Sig.	Partial Eta Squared	Noncent. Parameter	Observed Power[a]
Assessment	Sphericity Assumed	.162	3	.054	26.908	.000	.379	80.725	1.000
	Greenhouse-Geisser	.162	2.258	.072	26.908	.000	.379	60.769	1.000
	Huynh-Feldt	.162	2.441	.066	26.908	.000	.379	65.680	1.000
	Lower-bound	.162	1.000	.162	26.908	.000	.379	26.908	.999
Assessment * Track_Train	Sphericity Assumed	.008	3	.003	1.357	.259	.030	4.070	.354
	Greenhouse-Geisser	.008	2.258	.004	1.357	.263	.030	3.064	.304
	Huynh-Feldt	.008	2.441	.003	1.357	.262	.030	3.311	.317
	Lower-bound	.008	1.000	.008	1.357	.250	.030	1.357	.207
Error(Assessment)	Sphericity Assumed	.264	132	.002					
	Greenhouse-Geisser	.264	99.369	.003					
	Huynh-Feldt	.264	107.398	.002					
	Lower-bound	.264	44.000	.006					

a. Computed using alpha = .05

Tests of Between-Subjects Effects

Measure:MEASURE_1

Transformed Variable:Average

Source	Type III Sum of Squares	df	Mean Square	F	Sig.	Partial Eta Squared	Noncent. Parameter	Observed Power[a]
Intercept	45.323	1	45.323	2413.931	.000	.982	2413.931	1.000
Track_Train	.011	1	.011	.572	.454	.013	.572	.115
Error	.826	44	.019					

a. Computed using alpha = .05

3. Track_Train * Assessment

Measure:MEASURE_1

Track_Train	Assessment	Mean	Std. Error	95% Confidence Interval	
				Lower Bound	Upper Bound
.00	1	.568	.034	.500	.636
	2	.595	.025	.544	.645
	3	.628	.023	.582	.673
	4	.673	.022	.629	.717
1.00	1	.576	.017	.542	.609
	2	.632	.012	.607	.657
	3	.662	.011	.640	.685
	4	.671	.011	.649	.693

Tests of Within-Subjects Effects

Multivariate Tests[c]

Effect		Value	F	Hypothesis df	Error df	Sig.	Partial Eta Squared	Noncent. Parameter	Observed Power[b]
Assessment	Pillai's Trace	.578	19.148[a]	3.000	42.000	.000	.578	57.445	1.000
	Wilks' Lambda	.422	19.148[a]	3.000	42.000	.000	.578	57.445	1.000
	Hotelling's Trace	1.368	19.148[a]	3.000	42.000	.000	.578	57.445	1.000
	Roy's Largest Root	1.368	19.148[a]	3.000	42.000	.000	.578	57.445	1.000
Assessment * Track_Train	Pillai's Trace	.011	.161[a]	3.000	42.000	.922	.011	.484	.077
	Wilks' Lambda	.989	.161[a]	3.000	42.000	.922	.011	.484	.077
	Hotelling's Trace	.012	.161[a]	3.000	42.000	.922	.011	.484	.077
	Roy's Largest Root	.012	.161[a]	3.000	42.000	.922	.011	.484	.077

a. Exact statistic

b. Computed using alpha = .05

Within-Subjects Factors

Measure:MEASURE_1

Assessment	Dependent Variable
1	AI_incomp.1.00
2	AI_incomp.2.00
3	AI_incomp.3.00
4	AI_incomp.4.00

c. Design: Intercept + Track_Train
Within Subjects Design: Assessment

Measure:MEASURE_1

Source		Type III Sum of Squares	df	Mean Square	F	Sig.	Partial Eta Squared	Noncent. Parameter	Observed Power[a]
Assessment	Sphericity Assumed	.464	3	.155	23.251	.000	.346	69.752	1.000
	Greenhouse-Geisser	.464	2.436	.190	23.251	.000	.346	56.631	1.000
	Huynh-Feldt	.464	2.647	.175	23.251	.000	.346	61.556	1.000
	Lower-bound	.464	1.000	.464	23.251	.000	.346	23.251	.997
Assessment * Track_Train	Sphericity Assumed	.002	3	.001	.125	.945	.003	.374	.072
	Greenhouse-Geisser	.002	2.436	.001	.125	.917	.003	.304	.070
	Huynh-Feldt	.002	2.647	.001	.125	.929	.003	.330	.071
	Lower-bound	.002	1.000	.002	.125	.726	.003	.125	.064
Error(Assessment)	Sphericity Assumed	.878	132	.007					
	Greenhouse-Geisser	.878	107.170	.008					
	Huynh-Feldt	.878	116.490	.008					
	Lower-bound	.878	44.000	.020					

a. Computed using alpha = .05

Tests of Between-Subjects Effects

Measure:MEASURE_1

Transformed Variable:Average

Source	Type III Sum of Squares	df	Mean Square	F	Sig.	Partial Eta Squared	Noncent. Parameter	Observed Power[a]
Intercept	33.656	1	33.656	488.153	.000	.917	488.153	1.000
Track_Train	.015	1	.015	.216	.645	.005	.216	.074
Error	3.034	44	.069					

a. Computed using alpha = .05

3. Track_Train * Assessment

Measure:MEASURE_1

Track_Train	Assessment	Mean	Std. Error	95% Confidence Interval	
				Lower Bound	Upper Bound
.00	1	.460	.058	.343	.576
	2	.539	.058	.421	.657
	3	.585	.045	.494	.675
	4	.618	.033	.551	.685
1.00	1	.427	.029	.370	.485
	2	.508	.029	.450	.566
	3	.574	.022	.529	.618
	4	.602	.016	.568	.635

CPSIA information can be obtained
at www.ICGtesting.com
Printed in the USA
LVIW021431250113
317290LV00005B